billion
dollar
smile

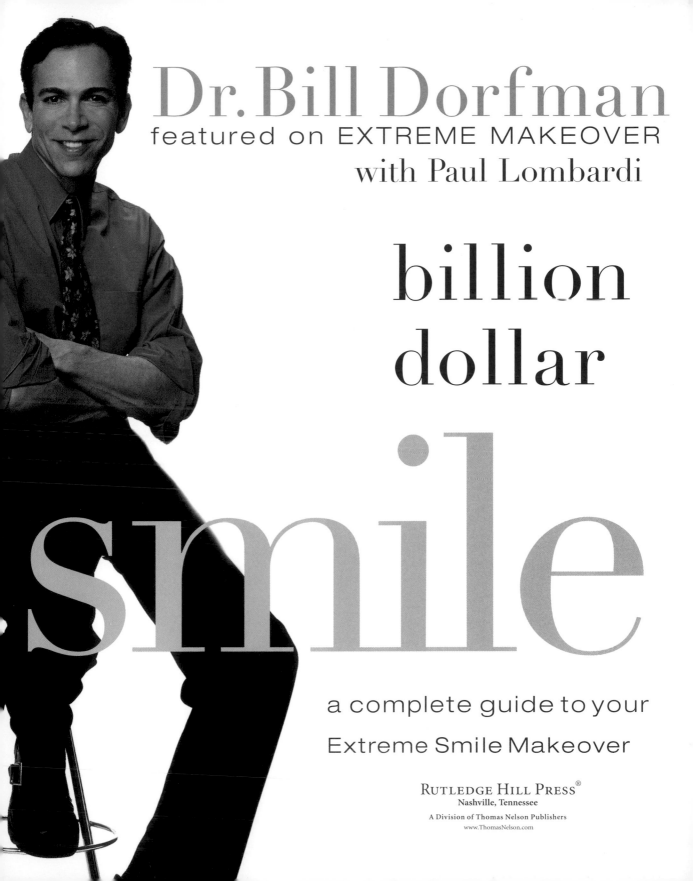

Dr. Bill Dorfman
featured on EXTREME MAKEOVER
with Paul Lombardi

billion
dollar
smile

a complete guide to your
Extreme Smile Makeover

RUTLEDGE HILL PRESS®
Nashville, Tennessee
A Division of Thomas Nelson Publishers
www.ThomasNelson.com

Published by Rutledge Hill Press, a Division of Thomas Nelson, Inc., P.O. Box 141000, Nashville, Tennessee 37214.

Rutledge Hill Press books may be purchased in bulk for educational, business, fundraising, or sales promotional use. For information, please e-mail SpecialMarkets@ThomasNelson.com.

The Smile Guide section is adapted from *Smile Guide* by Dr. Bill Dorfman, copyright © 1990, 2004 Discus Dental, Inc. All rights reserved. Used with permission.

The information in this book is for general knowledge only. Consult with your dentist or physician before undergoing any medical or dental procedures. Seek prompt dental care for any specific dental problem or concern.

Edited by Sara J. Henry

Text design: Bill Chiaravalle, Mark Mickel, Brand Navigation, LLC.

Smile Guide photography (pages 19–31): Trish O'Reilly

Smile Guide illustrations: Medart Media, Inc.

Library of Congress Cataloging-in-Publication Data

Dorfman, Bill, 1958–
    Billion dollar smile : a complete guide to your extreme smile makeover / Bill Dorfman with Paul Lombardi.
      p. cm.
    Includes index
    ISBN-13: 978-1-4016-0249-9 (trade paper)
    ISBN-10: 1-4016-0249-5 (trade paper)
    1. Dentistry—Aesthetic aspects. 2. Smiling. I. Lombardi, Paul. II. Title.
RK54.D67 2006
617.6—dc22   2006014508

Printed in the United States of America

06 07 08 09 10 — 5 4 3

In loving memory of my grandparents

and to Graham Dankworth, the son of Drs. Kim and Steve Dankworth,

and Dustin Wells, the son of my "best man," Dr. Dennis Wells

All of my proceeds from this book will be donated to the Dustin Wells Memorial Foundation, to the American Heart Association, and to the Garth Brooks Teammates for Kids Foundation to fund the Crown Council's Smiles for Life Foundation and the National Children's Dental Foundation. If you wish to help a child smile, please contact the National Children's Dental Foundation at www.tncdf.org or 800-559-9838. One hundred percent of your donation will go directly to providing dental care for children living in poverty.

—Dr. Bill Dorfman

contents

acknowledgments

I'd like to thank my family, friends, and mentors, who have given me love and support throughout my life. I owe the deepest gratitude to my parents, who are the best parents I could ever be blessed with; my siblings; my business partner and lifelong closest friend, Robert Hayman; my office (and everyday life) manager, Jill Ullman; my dental office employees; my coauthor, Paul Lombardi; my children, Anna, Charlotte, and Georgia; and my wife, Jennifer, the most amazing, beautiful, and loving woman in the world.

—Dr. Bill Dorfman

I would like to thank my good friend, the inspirational and unstoppable Bill Dorfman, and his girls for welcoming me into their family. And thank you, Bill, for creating my own Billion Dollar Smile!

I am forever grateful to my wonderful, warm partner, Jeff Soref; my loyal and supportive friends Andrew Kirtzman, Jack Stephenson, Alysa Wakin, Candy Knorr, Laura Maslow, and Ken Sunshine; and my loving family, especially my friend and gifted fellow writer, my brother Tom. You all give me a billion reasons to smile every day.

Bill and I both want to thank our visionary agent, Jan Miller; her associate literary agent, Annabelle Baxter; our generous publisher, Pamela Clements; our sharp editors, Jennifer Greenstein and Sara Henry; and our publicity powerhouses, Melanie Bryant, Paul Gendreau, and Nancy Iannios for making our book a reality.

—Paul Lombardi

introduction

The only thing that warms the heart as much as a beautiful song is a beautiful smile.

—GARTH BROOKS

Before you read another word, walk over to a mirror. Now say "cheese." What do you see? Is your smile dingy and dark—or healthy and bright? Is it a Billion Dollar Smile?

Are you completely happy with your smile? Do you feel self-conscious when you laugh or when you meet someone for the first time? As the saying goes, you have only one chance to make a good first impression. Your smile is the first thing people notice about you. Who can resist a pearly white smile?

I'm here to help you make your smile makeover a reality—an affordable reality. You'll have to maintain it, but your new smile will never go out of style.

Mike Myers may have made crooked, discolored teeth funny in his *Austin Powers* movies, but in real life bad teeth are nothing to laugh about. Looks do count in today's increasingly image-conscious world, and an unattractive smile is simply no longer acceptable.

Society judges a book by its cover, so you need to look your best. Even if *you* don't care what you look like, other people do. It's a scientific fact, a part of nature, that human beings respond favorably to a nice smile.

According to the American Academy of Cosmetic Dentistry, 99.7 percent of Americans believe a smile is an important social asset—and 96 percent believe an attractive smile makes you more appealing to members of the opposite sex. Three-quarters of adults feel an unattractive smile can hurt your chances for career success.

Like they say with the lottery, you gotta be in it to win it. You have to play the game. Life is hard enough, and a bright, beautiful smile can help open doors and hearts. You'll be amazed at how much more confident you'll feel with a Billion Dollar Smile. As the English naturalist John Ray once said, "Beauty is power; a smile is its sword."

And you know what I say to all those critics out there who dismiss cosmetic surgery as superficial? So what? It is superficial! But so are many of the things in our lives: clothing, haircuts, cars, and houses. If you want to do something about your appearance and you can, then go for it! I'm not suggesting you take it to the extreme—unless you have significant dental problems—but if a new smile will make you feel more confident and attractive, you owe it to yourself to go out and get one.

I practice in the Beverly Hills area, so it's no surprise that many of my patients have "gone under the knife" for plastic surgery. But they all say that even after plastic surgery, their new look isn't complete without a beautiful smile. The smile brings the whole package together—like the cherry on a sundae.

Dentistry is going through a revolution. Don't settle for simply getting by without cavities! Taking good care of your teeth—brushing them, flossing them, and refraining from using them to open bottles—does not guarantee a nice smile. But I can help you have healthy teeth *and* a dazzling, jaw-dropping smile.

If you're completely comfortable with your smile and what others think of your appearance and you feel no need to upgrade your smile, great. Good for you. Luckily, for the rest of us there's cosmetic dentistry. You'll be blown away by the advances in dental science and the choices now available.

We created *Billion Dollar Smile* to be the extreme, end-all guide for anyone, dentists included, who wants to create a beautiful smile and understand the impact that a smile can have on our lives. *Billion Dollar Smile* will show you ways to brighten your smile for the price of a new dress or a new suit. You might wear that outfit only once or twice, but you'll wear that new smile every day for the rest of your life.

This book is also a "how-to" book—how to design your own Billion Dollar Smile. For some, it could be as simple as a quick whitening and contouring appointment. For others, it may involve surgery.

With before and after photographs and amusing and touching stories from my patients, including celebrities and *Extreme Makeover* participants, *Billion Dollar Smile* will educate you so you can determine what may work best for you. You will learn what to ask for at the dentist's office and will become fluent in "dentalese."

This book will serve as a "mouth manual." With pictures matching face types to teeth types, we will help you articulate your vision for your new face. The possibilities are endless. After reading this book you will have the knowledge and the courage to fix your grin and maximize your potential, both in the boardroom and the bedroom!

Of course, you're probably wondering how much your Billion Dollar Smile will cost. Costs for procedures can vary depending on where you live. Just like food and housing, you'll pay a lot more for cosmetic dentistry in a big city or an expensive suburb than in other areas. You'll also pay more for some procedures than for others. You and your dentist will decide what works best for you and your budget. In some cases, a more moderately priced procedure can produce excellent results. I often stress that "less can be best." This book will help you navigate the options available and familiarize you with their relative affordability so you and your dentist can make an informed decision.

When my coauthor, Paul Lombardi, first approached me about writing this book, he asked, "Who better to lead consumers by the hand through the many choices in cosmetic dentistry than America's dentist?" You may know me as that dentist who gets hugs from his patients every week on ABC's *Extreme Makeover*. In addition, I have more than twenty years of experience in cosmetic dentistry. I also founded Discus Dental, the largest direct dental sales company in the world, and invented or coinvented several innovative dental products used by millions all over the world, including the whiteners Nite White, Day White, and ZOOM! and the breath control system BreathRx. Recently, Discus Dental purchased BriteSmile, an in-office whitening system that is similar to the ZOOM! system.

I consider myself lucky because ever since I was three years old I knew what I wanted to be when I grew up—a dentist! Pretty geeky, huh? Well, sometimes, geeks get lucky. One day I was examining the teeth of an A-list movie star that *People* magazine once named "Sexiest Man of the Year." A little boy peeked into the treatment room, and in a shy, quiet voice with his hands behind his back, he said, "I know you." When the movie star spoke up, the little fellow said, "Not you!" and pointed to me and said, "You! You're Dr. Bill the dentist!"

It's pretty cool getting recognized by a kid, but it took the supermodel Cindy Crawford to really make an impact on me. I'm accustomed to meeting celebrities, because I treat many of them at my practice, but Cindy has always made my knees wobble. After years of admiring her from a distance, I finally saw her at a party. In the flesh! I took a few deep breaths and finally got up the nerve to go over and say hello. I made my way across the crowded room and just as I said, "Hi, I'm Bill . . ." she interrupted and screamed, "Oh, my God! Dr. Dorfman, I love you! I watch your show all the time!" Now that's something to smile about.

Like many things, it all goes back to my childhood. When I was just two years old, I fell down and hit my baby teeth so hard that they were knocked up *into* my gums. That was no fun. Over the next few years, I underwent several intensive surgeries to ensure my adult teeth would grow in normally. Ironically, instead of becoming scared of dentistry, I became fascinated with it. I was kind of like that elf kid in the animated Christmas special *Rudolph the Red-Nosed Reindeer*, the one who wants to be a dentist when all the other elves just want to make toys. When every other kid wanted to be a fireman, I wanted to be a dentist. Seriously though, it was through the life-altering experience of my accident and recovery that I learned that a smile is nothing to take for granted.

A beautiful smile can be one of your greatest assets. At a recent dental conference, thousands of dentists were asked what fee they would demand in exchange for their upper front teeth. The average answer was more than one million dollars. That shouldn't be surprising. Throughout history, people have noticed and appreciated a great smile, whether on Mona Lisa or Julia Roberts. Miguel de Cervantes said in *Don Quixote* that every tooth in a man's head is more valuable than a diamond.

My goal is to help you make your smile sparkle like diamonds. I feel incredibly blessed knowing I make people's lives better. And as the dentist on *Extreme Makeover*, I've been fortunate to have the opportunity to improve many smiles.

People always wonder how I got my role on the show. Well, as they say in Hollywood, it's all about who you know. And in Hollywood you never know who knows whom! One of my patients, Jennifer Cole Fenton, had been a game show hostess on a show produced by Howard Schultz. When Howard and Jennifer were chatting about his new project, *Extreme Makeover*, Jennifer (who should be an agent) told him to check out her boss, Beverly Hills plastic surgeon Dr. Garth Fisher, for whom she worked as an assistant between TV gigs. So Howard and his team met Dr. Fisher, and that's how they found their first makeover expert.

The producers already had a dentist in mind, but Jennifer and my good friend Garth suggested that they also talk to me. The producers called me and told me they were interested in meeting immediately because they needed to make a decision that evening. Everything needs to be done yesterday in TV! Unfortunately I had a number of patients that day, so I couldn't go over to meet them in person. However, I did have a demo reel—a compilation of all the TV interviews I've done over the years. In lieu of an actual audition, I sent my reel over to the producers, and once they saw that I was comfortable in front of the camera, they called me back and told me that I'd landed the job.

I must admit that at first I was a bit hesitant about joining the "extreme team" of doctors, because initially I was afraid the show might exploit the participants and turn them into "reality TV victims." But I met with Howard, the creator, and Jacqui Pitman, his executive producing partner, and sensed that their hearts were in the right place. The producers expressed supreme kindness, compassion, and concern for the participants. So I took a leap of faith and virtually put my reputation and the future of Discus Dental in the hands of Lighthearted Entertainment and ABC.

Taping the show turned out to be a lot of fun, though when we first started I really had no idea what the program was all about. I definitely had no idea that it was going to air nationally. Everything seemed so low key; I thought that it would just be shown locally on a small ABC affiliate.

But as thrilled as I was to be part of this exciting new show, I was a little frustrated after the pilot because all I got to do was ZOOM! whiten the patients' teeth. As you'll discover as you read this book, cosmetic dentistry has so much more to offer. So in an attempt to show how incomplete a makeover is without a killer smile, I sent my most dramatic "before" and "after" dental photos to the producers. Along with the pictures I included a thank you note saying how much I enjoyed being on the show and suggesting that if we got picked up for a full season, cosmetic dentistry could add a whole new dimension to the makeovers. I don't think any of us, including the patients, were prepared for the impact these smile makeovers would have on our lives.

Before *Extreme Makeover*, dentists got a pretty bad rap in the media and were not represented very well in pop culture. Remember the Nazi dentist in the film *Marathon Man* or Steve Martin's sadistic turn as a dentist in *Little Shop of Horrors*? This is what we were up against! *Extreme Makeover* made dentistry the hero week after week on prime time television. For that, my profession and I will be eternally grateful to the production team of *Extreme Makeover*, especially Howard, Jacqui, Chuck Bangert, Lou Gorfain, Janis Biewend, Andrea Schwartzberg, Julie Laughlin, Marla Brodsky, Jason Hoffman, and Andrea Wong, along with everyone else at ABC.

Some of the makeover stories you're about to read might make you cry; some will make you laugh. These are real people we worked with, some of whom have become very good friends of mine. And although the doctors get the credit, I applaud the patients. They are the real heroes.

We all have something we don't like about our bodies. Maybe it's your nose, your ears, your behind, your thighs, or your smile. As hard as it is for us to admit that to ourselves, it is even harder to admit it to others. The patients on *Extreme Makeover* exposed themselves, in the most vulnerable way I could imagine, to millions of viewers all over the world. Their courage, in turn, touched others—those who may have felt trapped in bodies they didn't know how to change. I believe the show empowered people to say that it's okay to want to change yourself for the better.

But it's important to understand that the message of *Extreme Makeover* is not that you have to have plastic surgery or cosmetic dentistry to lead a full, rich life. The message is that if you are unhappy with your appearance and it is impairing your confidence or your health, you can do something about it.

I hope that *Billion Dollar Smile* will move and inspire you with the stories of patients whose new smiles gave them a new outlook on life. At the same time, this book will walk you through all the cosmetic dental choices available and present you with innovative options that will leave you smiling from ear to ear. Through a thoughtful marriage of art and science, I will help *you* create your own custom-made Billion Dollar Smile.

billion
dollar
smile

a smile speaks volumes

1

razzle dazzle 'em

THE BENEFITS OF
COSMETIC DENTISTRY

Like it or not, it's a sad but true reality that people *do* judge a book by its cover. You get only one chance to make a first impression.

Cosmetic dentistry offers both physical and psychological benefits. An unattractive mouth can make you miserable, but a dazzling smile can improve your self-esteem. A smile can also speak volumes about your health, how you take care of yourself, and how old you look.

Now it is time for you to learn how to capitalize on your smile. You will be amazed to read true accounts about people who used to lead sad, misunderstood lives: beautiful people cursed with less-than-beautiful smiles that didn't reflect and radiate who they were on the inside. Maybe you, too, feel ashamed of your teeth. Are you afraid to smile, afraid to really live and express your true self?

a life transformed: DeShanté Hall

DeShanté Hall is the heart of this chapter—and the whole book for that matter. As one of my *Extreme Makeover* miracles, she personifies the *Billion Dollar Smile* philosophy and humanizes society's conviction that looks do matter. A beautiful smile says, "I'm attractive, I'm confident, I'm in control, and I'm healthy."

BEFORE THE MAKEOVER

As you'll see in the "before" photos, before the Extreme Team worked its magic, DeShanté had an asymmetrical face. She was born with a cleft lip and palate, which is an opening in the lip and roof of the mouth that can cause dental, speech, and other problems—and she was also missing front teeth. The result was a huge gap in her smile.

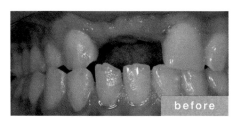
before

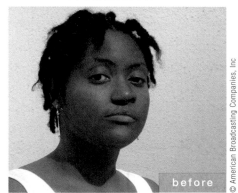
before

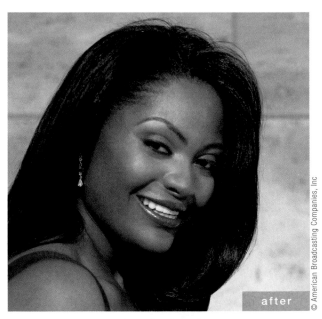
after

DeShanté Hall had a cleft palate and missing teeth. Her Extreme Makeover included a nose job, corrective lip surgery, a permanently cemented porcelain bridge, and porcelain veneers.

DeShanté's parents did their best to help their daughter, but after several childhood surgeries failed to do the trick, her emotional scars ran just as deep as her physical ones. She was teased so badly that she didn't even want to leave the house. And forget about smiling. DeShanté opened her mouth only when she absolutely had to. She suffered as a teenager as well: no dating, no boys, no self-esteem. But DeShanté wasn't a quitter.

She couldn't afford to have corrective cosmetic surgery, and she was sick of the pain her appearance burdened her with every waking minute of her life. But DeShanté found joy attending church, and she says her Extreme Makeover was an answer to prayer.

When I met DeShanté, I think I was more excited about helping her than she was about getting help. I was so eager to be a part of this young woman's transformation that I could barely sleep the night before.

DESHANTÉ'S NEW SMILE

DeShanté wanted to make her face more symmetrical. That meant a nose job, corrective lip surgery, and most importantly, new teeth. Her lip was collapsed and new teeth were needed to give her lip support so one side wouldn't cave in. She was also missing two upper front teeth.

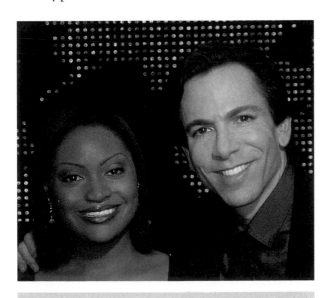

One year after her Extreme Makeover, DeShanté Hall appeared with me on *Larry King Live.*

I used a permanently cemented porcelain bridge and porcelain veneers (more on these later) to replace the missing teeth. Because of her cleft palate, there was no bone, so she could not have teeth implants. When I was finally through, after hours and hours working on her mouth, DeShanté was in tears. I was worried she might be in pain, but she said she was crying because she was so happy. At age twenty-two, DeShanté's new life had just begun.

DeShanté's new face in the "after"

photo shows that the beautiful person on the outside has finally caught up with the beautiful person on the inside!

I wanted to share DeShanté's personal and poignant story because her uplifting account can inspire you to change your life too. While you may not need work as extensive as DeShanté's, even minor cosmetic procedures can make an enormous difference in your smile, your appearance—and your attitude.

Several months after she went home, I received a very moving letter from DeShanté. After thanking me for transforming her smile and ultimately her life, she wrote:

> It's amazing how differently people treat you when you fit into their ideal of beauty. It's a bittersweet thing. I've always been this person. However few people took the time to get to know me. Now people that wouldn't even make eye contact with me have so much to say.

Now DeShanté says she smiles all the time. And for the first time in her life men are pursuing her! Her new mantra is "There are so many men out there and so little time. What's a girl to do?"

Well, this girl finally picked a guy. DeShanté tells me she's very happy with a wonderful guy she knew before her makeover. She says, "More than anything, I am now more confident and more approachable. Some of the issues I used to have to deal with before made me unapproachable. I was angry, embarrassed, and upset and people sensed that energy."

DeShanté says her boyfriend claims he was interested in her before the makeover, but DeShanté wasn't open to love then. She was too busy being down on herself. But with her new look and smile, she's happier with herself, which allows her to be more receptive and not afraid of rejection.

Having a guy in her life who thinks she is beautiful is a dream come true for DeShanté. A close second is having her little niece, Leilani, call her beautiful. DeShanté knew she was ready to begin her new life empowered and humanized by her Billion Dollar Smile.

That's the kind of smile power I can help you tap into. Whether your goal is being attractive, improving your career, or just feeling better about yourself, a new smile can and will make a dramatic difference in your life. Trust me, I know what I'm doing. I have even had patients insist on having "Dental care from Dr. Bill until I die" written into their divorce contracts.

IN DESHANTÉ'S OWN WORDS

DeShanté Hall articulates what it's like to experience life as a "before and after" person in a poem she graciously shared for this book.

IT'S ME

I've spent so much time
Running from myself
Warring against the cards I was dealt
From the rise and fall of my dress size
To the genetics that have given me
this blessing in disguise
But I have come to realize
I'm a woman strong and complete
No longer avoiding my reality
But embracing all I am meant to be
I am set aside
Standing solely acceptingly

In the midst of all the Lord has planned for me
I stand
Faithfully gracefully
An inspiration
Still constantly improving
Now
Stepping confidently to the other side of insecurity
I have made it through still holding on to love
Completely happily enjoying me

A new smile will make your package more complete. DeShanté's mom articulates it quite well. She says that before her makeover DeShanté was beautiful, but now with her Billion Dollar Smile, she is gorgeous.

Psychologists say you communicate just as much with your mouth as you do with your body—and that smiling is one form of body language that can make you more attractive. It's no surprise that studies show that a smile is generally perceived as more attractive than a pout; in other words, you are more approachable and desirable when you look happy. And it all goes uphill from there. Studies also suggest that people believe those who are physically attractive have other positive traits as well.

Rumi, the thirteenth-century Persian poet, told the story of a little girl who lost her smile. She wakes up sad one morning and turns a city gray because only her smile can bring out the sun. When she smiles again, the sun shines once more in all its glory. As for that other girl who found her true self through her smile makeover, DeShanté Hall continues to inspire me to help people transform their smiles and their lives. I hope her story will inspire you as well, as you learn more about how you can create your own Billion Dollar Smile.

design
the smile
of your
dreams

2

a gallery of smiles

SELECTING YOUR BILLION DOLLAR SMILE

A smile is a work of art. But sometimes even masterpieces can use a little tweaking. We'll start with the smile you were born with and make it more dazzling, while maintaining its unique character and personality.

With elective cosmetic dentistry, there is nothing medically wrong with your teeth. You have no major oral health problems and you haven't been in an accident. Your gums are healthy, you have no cavities, and your teeth are functioning properly. You simply want a cosmetic improvement, perhaps to look younger, healthier, sexier, and more attractive. Nothing wrong with that!

What I call the broken smile is another story. A broken smile is a smile that needs to be repaired for health and functional reasons. But while you're at it, you might as well take the plunge and have cosmetic improvements too!

This chapter is all about aesthetics. (We'll explore the dental procedures in Chapter 4.) The following pages will help you decide which smile best suits your features, your personality, and in a word, *you*. Some women tear celebrity photos out of magazines and bring them to their hairdressers and say, "Make me look like Jennifer Aniston." Well, *Billion Dollar Smile* can do that for teeth.

You can take this book with you to the dentist's office, open it up to this chapter, and point to the smile you want. It will be a great tool for your cosmetic dentist, just as it helps your hairdresser when you take a photo along to show what you want. Obviously, creating a smile is a lot more complicated than cutting hair, but you get the idea.

There's the medical and functional aspect of dentistry, and there's the artistry. I may be a dentist, but make no mistake—I am also an artist. My drill isn't exactly a paintbrush, but you'll be amazed how a dentist can create a gleaming, attractive smile for any face, including yours.

By shaping your teeth we can highlight your face's best features and downplay your less appealing characteristics. Realize that your goal, however, should not be perfection. If teeth are too even, too straight, or too white, you will end up looking artificial. Nothing in nature is ever perfect or perfectly symmetrical, and teeth are no exception to that rule.

It's the same thing with plastic surgery. The best surgeries are the ones that elicit compliments such as: "You look great, really healthy, and well rested"—not "Wow, your last surgery turned out really well!" A fresh, new smile can do that for you. And if you're looking great, chances are you're feeling pretty great as well.

collaborating with your dentist

Often, people will come to my office with a preconceived notion of what they want. They bring in pictures of celebrities, models, or relatives for me to use as a reference. Or I ask them to give me a picture of themselves from a time in their life when they liked their smile and go from there.

One of my favorite patients, the Hollywood legend Esther Williams, brought in pictures taken when she was in her twenties and asked to look like that again. Esther, by the way, is just as graceful, classy, and beautiful today as ever. It was an honor to create a dazzling smile to complement her dazzling beauty. More about that later!

Years ago, I wrote a book called *The Smile Guide* (portions of an updated version appear at the end of this chapter) so patients could select the teeth of their choosing. I wrote it because patients had a hard time finding pictures in magazines where you could actually see every tooth displayed in a smile. I wanted a clear, anatomically correct book of smile styles so patients could go through the book and explain exactly what they wanted to their dentist, and the dentist could, in turn, use the book to communicate to the dental laboratory and the technicians who make the teeth exactly what the new teeth should look like.

This was revolutionary in dentistry because there had never been a book like it. Whether you are revamping your smile purely for cosmetic reasons or because it is "broken," the most important aspect of creating a new smile is for the cosmetic dentist to really listen to what the patient wants and then deliver.

Yes, it should be a collaboration and, yes, I believe that cosmetic dentists (good ones, anyway) are artists who have their own vision. But you're the one who has to look at yourself in the mirror every day. While you should be open to your dentist's suggestions, if you're adamant about a certain smile, then you should have the last word.

A lot of aesthetic dentists create teeth using certain parameters, like the golden proportion, an industry-wide recommendation on length and width of teeth. But my style is to stay away from strict rules and numbers and work more like an artist. To me every smile is like a blank palette, and my goal is to create the most harmonious and aesthetically pleasing result possible. And because every face, every smile, every individual is unique, rules are not steadfast.

A smile isn't just about teeth shapes. It is also about the position of the teeth: how the uppers are positioned against the lowers, where the gum position is, and how the lips fall against the teeth and frame the smile.

I heard a great analogy once: Your mouth is like a theater—your two front teeth are the lead actors and the teeth surrounding them are the supporting cast members. The smile is the stage and the lips are the curtains.

If you create a beautiful smile with insufficiently short lips, so that far too much gum shows, it's not a pretty smile, no matter how beautiful the teeth are.

Often the best place to start is to first look at what you currently have. Typically, you are born with your most natural smile, and you and your dentist don't want to deviate too much from that—just enhance it.

facing your face

Let me help you decide which smile works for you.

My good friend and mentor, Dr. Jeff Golub-Evans from New York City, is a preeminent "smile designer." I agree with his philosophy of masking or minimizing the negative features on a face and maximizing the positive features. He says it's about matching the smile to the entire face and ultimately to the whole person. Here are illustrations of how a smile can influence the perceived shape of your face. (Note: The photos in this section have been digitally altered for illustration purposes.)

First, identify your face shape. Is your face oval, long, round, heart-shaped, or square?

OVAL FACE

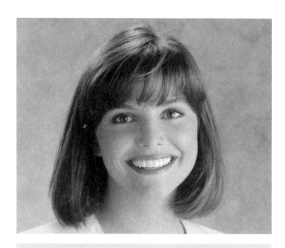

The oval face is usually considered the most desirable by Western society.

If your face is oval, then you have your pick of the litter, so to speak. This face shape has long been considered to be one of the most perfect in Western society. Pretty much any smile works because an oval face is so well proportioned. So go to town! Big teeth, little teeth, long or short— an oval face can handle it. (The trick is to make other face shapes look more oval in appearance.)

LONG FACE

For a long face, you'll want a more even, horizontal row of teeth to offset the vertical or upright appearance of the face. Smaller front teeth are probably a better choice, because long teeth will only accentuate your face shape. In addition, the smile should be made broader or wider by bulking out the molars and premolars.

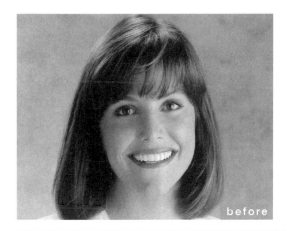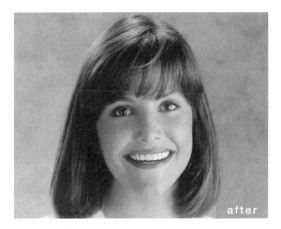

The long face can be made to appear shorter by an optical illusion created by teeth. A broader smile and shorter front teeth help achieve this effect.

ROUND FACE

You want your smile to complement your face and enhance your features, and a smile with longer, more vertically shaped teeth will enhance a round face. The key to doing this is to lengthen the front teeth. One trick I like is to make the two front teeth just a little longer than the ones next to them.

QUESTIONS TO ASK YOURSELF WHILE SHOPPING FOR YOUR NEW SMILE:

> Does this smile suit my personality?
> Does this smile complement my face?
> Does this smile say what I want it to say?

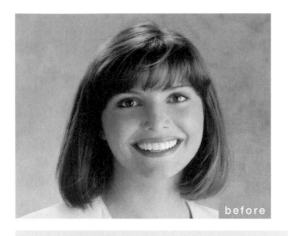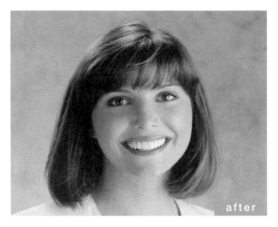

The round face can be made to appear longer with the appropriate teeth. An ideal smile design lengthens the front teeth and even makes the two upper front teeth a little longer than the ones next to them, creating a vertical stripe on the face.

HEART-SHAPED FACE

A heart-shaped face means the lower part of the face is more elongated. So the same thing applies here as for the long face: You'll want an even, horizontal row of smaller teeth, because long teeth will only accentuate your face shape. The goal here is to minimize the chin and enhance the width of the mouth.

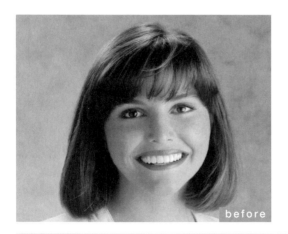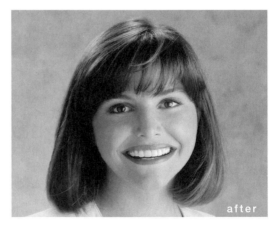

The heart-shaped face combines the features of the oval face in the top two-thirds and the long face in the lower one-third. The goal in creating the optimal design for this face is to minimize the chin by flattening the front teeth and widening the smile to create a horizontal stripe on the face.

SQUARE FACE

And last but not least for all you "squares" out there: Thanks to Cameron Diaz and Kirsten Dunst, it's now hip to be square. So be proud of your face and show it off with rectangular-shaped teeth that are a little longer.

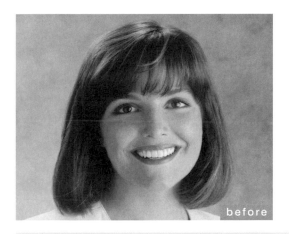 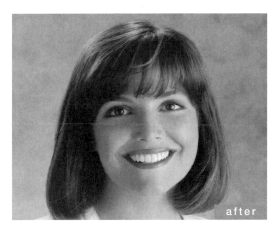

The square face has come into vogue as the current image of androgynous beauty. To accentuate the square face, add a little length to the front teeth, creating a slightly longer appearance.

what type of smile suits you?

Once you've identified the shape of your face, you need to think about the type of smile you want. Smiles can say a lot about a person. They can reveal a wealth of information about who you are. There are carefree happy smiles, goofy smiles, sexy smiles, healthy smiles, mysterious smiles, anxious smiles, mischievous smiles, innocent smiles, young smiles, mature smiles, evil smiles, and even sad smiles.

Cosmetic dentists cannot, of course, create a personality. Your smile will reflect whatever it is you're feeling inside. I can, however, help you shape your image. For example, if you want attributes such as a young smile, a mature smile, a feminine smile, or a masculine smile, you can have the shape of your teeth contoured to reflect those attributes.

What your smile reveals is up to you.

YOUTHFUL SMILE

A youthful smile is an innocent, happy smile. It is also a smile that should only be seen on a younger person. I understand that "younger" is a subjective word. People are living longer, healthier lives and looking better than ever, but discretion is sorely needed in some areas.

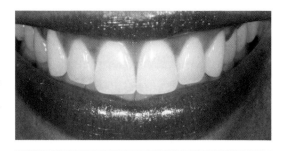

Youthful smile.

If you want to appear younger, then you don't want an even row of teeth. A more youthful smile means the teeth don't look ground down or sawed off. And a youthful smile shows at least three millimeters of teeth while speaking. (To assess this, I usually have my patients count from sixty-one to sixty-six and observe how much tooth is displayed.) The upper central incisors (two front teeth) should be slightly longer than the lateral incisors (the teeth next to the two front teeth). Younger teeth tend to be bigger teeth as well, because as we age our lips drop and cover more of our smile. A youthful-looking smile can often be achieved through veneers, bonding, or simply reshaping. (Chapter 4 has more details on these procedures.)

A young smile also is a whiter smile. It is fresh and not yet stained by years of stain-inducing foods and beverages.

MATURE SMILE

Two things can make a smile look older.

Have you ever heard that expression "long in the tooth," meaning older? As we get older our spines become shorter, and many times our gums recede as well. When our gums recede, more tooth surface is exposed and therefore our teeth appear longer. This "long in the tooth" look is not a good look for

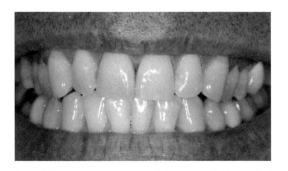

Mature smile.

anyone, especially when the newly exposed root surface is a different color or texture than the tooth. Ironically, as I mentioned earlier, our lips also drop as we age, so you might not see the gum recession unless you lift your lip.

Conversely, people who grind their teeth—whether during the day or night, or both—can wear their teeth down to short little stubs.

There is a happy medium. A mouth full of long, short, or age-inappropriate teeth isn't the best look for a mature smile. The best mature smile is just that: mature. The teeth are not too short or too long and tend to be even across the smile line. They are slightly more squared off and straighter in appearance than a younger smile. It's more handsome than cute, and this smile is appealing on mature women as well as mature men.

Mature smiles should be a more natural shade of white than younger smiles. Extremely white teeth look fake on a more mature face; a more muted shade of white works better.

FEMININE SMILE

They say a woman can get what she wants by "flashing her pearly whites." A feminine smile is bright, soft, and beguiling. How do you achieve this? Not unlike a feminine-looking body, a feminine-looking smile is all about curves. Teeth can be created or contoured with edges that are more rounded and softer looking.

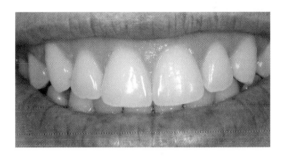

Feminine smile.

A pretty smile is the best accessory you can give yourself. When done right, it goes with absolutely everything!

MASCULINE SMILE

A man's smile should be charming and disarming at the same time. The teeth should be more angular than a woman's, and the central incisors should appear square, strong, and more powerful than the lateral incisors.

Masculine teeth should be white but not

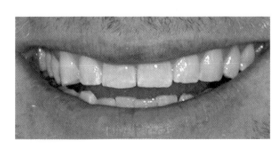

Masculine smile.

blindingly white, and the length should complement the face shape.

SAY CHEESE! HOW TO SMILE FOR THE CAMERA

Are you ever surprised when you see yourself in photographs? Do you wonder, "Who the heck is that?" Perhaps you think, "That looks kind of like me but it can't be!" It happens to all of us. Except maybe Paris Hilton, who seems to have been born posing for the camera. Just like everything else in life, smiling is an art, and I'll now share some tips on how to maximize your smile power and emphasize your good features:

Be real. A fake smile can be seen a mile away. Smile like you mean it! Even if you find yourself posing with your least favorite uncle whose breath smells worse than a swamp, a strained smile will be apparent. The camera doesn't lie.

Think ahead. Remember, smiles say a lot. Ask yourself what you want to say in a photo. Do you want to look sexy, smart, confident, mysterious, happy-go-lucky, dreamy, content? It sounds counterintuitive, but to present a smile that looks natural you might have to present a "premeditated" smile to get the result you're after.

Relax! The trick is to be as comfortable and relaxed as possible when you smile. Easier said than done when someone's pointing a camera at your head! You can tell when someone is radiating an honest-to-goodness real smile. Those types of people smile not only with their mouth but with their eyes, too.

Try a fake laugh. Ironically, when in doubt, the best way to make a warm "real" smile is to force a contained "fake" laugh. Most professional models give a muted chuckle when they smile for the camera.

Practice. This may sound vain and ridiculous, but it works very well. Practice smiling in front of a mirror. See how big a smile you can get away with before the crow's feet start to show. Do that several times until you get a feel for how wide a smile that is. Do you show too much gum? Practice controlling your lips and get to know your smile. What are its strengths and weaknesses? Is this the smile you think best represents you? Ideally, you would like the bottom of your upper lip to just touch the area where your upper front teeth meet the gums and for your lower lip to *not* cover the upper teeth (see the youthful smile on page 14).

Enlist a friend. Like Alicia Silverstone's character in the movie *Clueless,* some of us don't trust the mirror, so have a friend take pictures of you trying on different smiles. You can always return the favor. Take turns taking pictures and compare shots. Find one you like and practice smiling that smile on cue. Say cheese! When you get your Billion Dollar Smile, you won't have to worry about as many limitations. You'll be so proud of your new smile that you'll want to show it off everywhere you go!

the smile guide

One of the biggest obstacles between you and your Billion Dollar Smile is communication. You can consider this section as a type of dictionary to help you and your dentist speak the same language.

Way back in 1989, I started to see more and more patients in my practice who wanted to improve their smiles but either did not know what they wanted their new smiles to look like or could not explain their desired changes to me. After I was satisfied we had a mutual understanding, I then had the challenge of trying to explain this vision to my lab technician.

There are a variety of dental procedures available to improve the aesthetics of your smile, such as porcelain veneers, crowns, bonding, implants, cosmetic contouring, and removable appliances. Typically any one or combination of these procedures, along with tooth whitening, can be used to give you the smile of which you have always dreamed.

In the following pages you will see an abbreviated reprint of my first book, *The Smile Guide.* As you leaf through it, choose two or three smile styles that you believe would suit you and discuss these with your dentist. The first part of the Smile Guide (pages 19–31) shows full-face photographs of different smile styles, and the second part (pages 32–37) contains thirty-six diagrams of the most naturally occurring smile styles.

All the photographs and diagrams focus on the six upper front teeth because these vary the most from patient to patient. Although you may want to have Cindy Crawford's teeth, there may be limiting factors that would prevent your dentist from being able to do this for you. These include but are not limited to

> Alignment of your existing teeth
> Skeletal position of your jaws
> Contour of your gums and lips

VARIATIONS DEPICTED INCLUDE:

Central incisors

square	square oval	oval

Lateral incisors

square	square oval	oval

Canines

square	oval	pointed

As you review the diagrams beginning on page 32, you will observe the following patterns. There are six drawings per page. In the first three diagrams only the shape of the canines is altered. The last three smile styles are identical to the first three, except that the lateral incisors are shorter than the central incisors. Also note that for the most natural designs, the lateral incisor should always be the same as or more rounded than the central incisor.

As you look through the series of photos beginning on page 19, you will notice that in the beginning of the series, where the teeth are more square, there are more men, and as the teeth become rounder, toward the end of the series, there are more women. This is because square, even incisors are typically recognized as a masculine trait, while rounder oval teeth are interpreted as a softer, more feminine feature.

So, if you want the most bang for your dentistry buck, show this Smile Guide to your dentist and together the two of you can design the smile of your dreams.

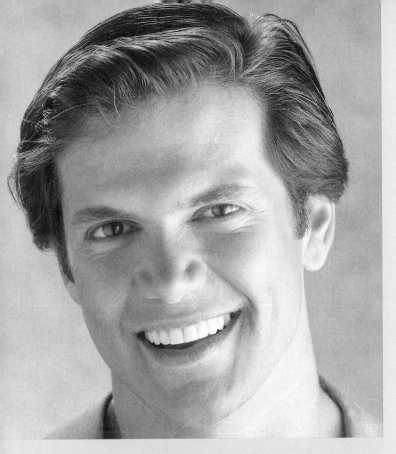

style no. 21
see page 33

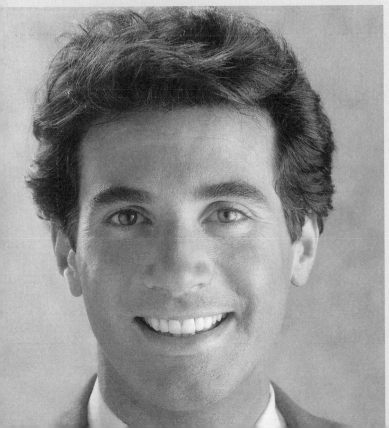

style no. 22
see page 33

19

style no. 15
see page 32

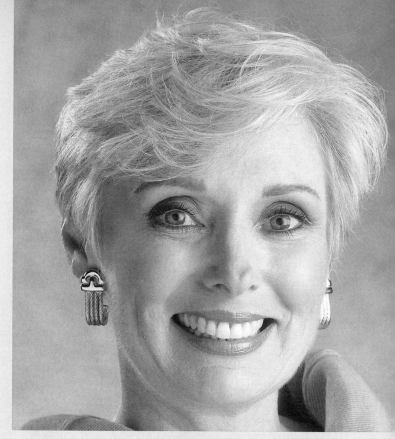

style no. 16
see page 32

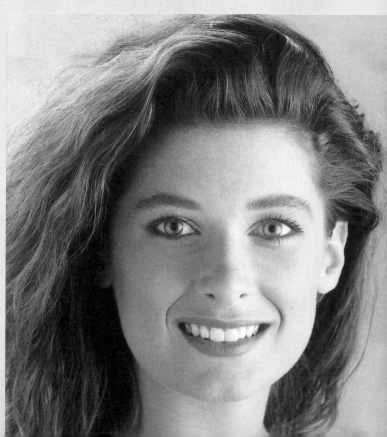

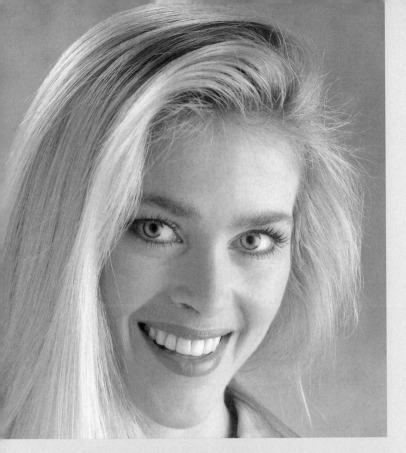

style no. 21
see page 33

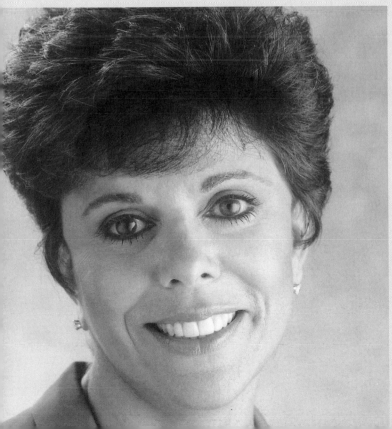

style no. 22
see page 33

style no. 24
see page 33

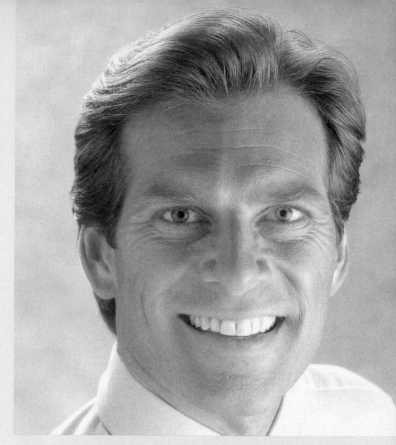

style no. 25
see page 33

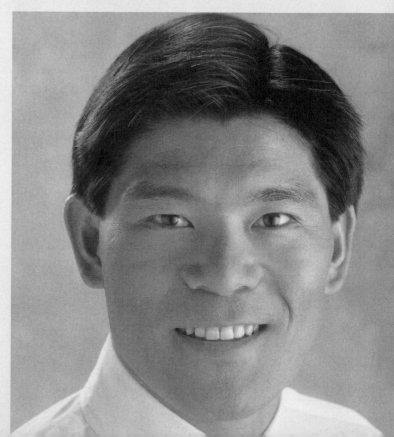

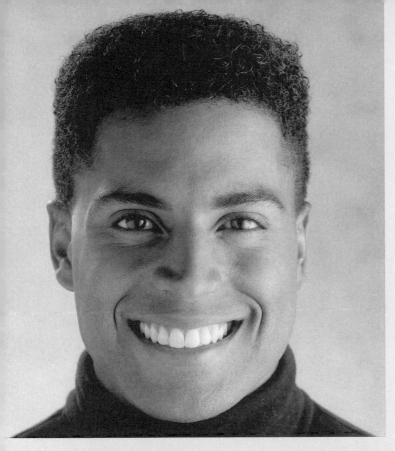

style no. 26
see page 33

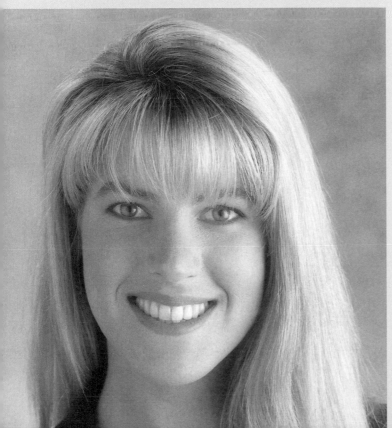

style no. 31
see page 34

style no. 33
see page 34

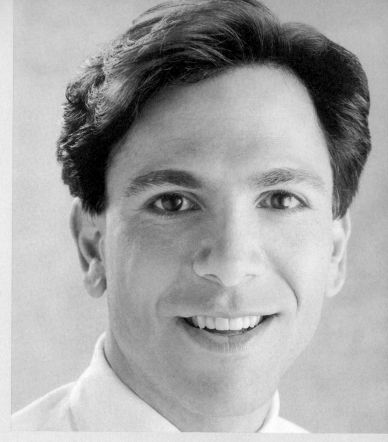

style no. 35
see page 34

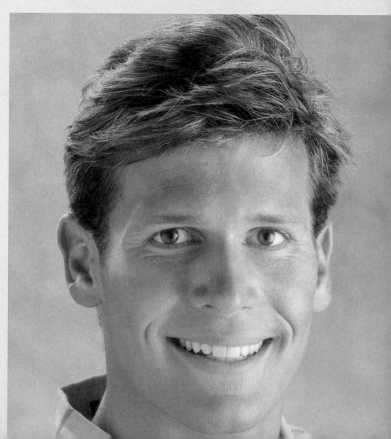

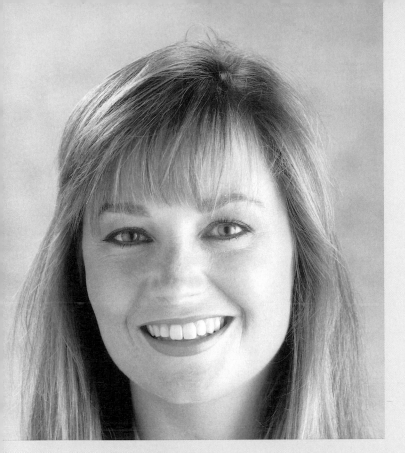

style no. 36

see page 34

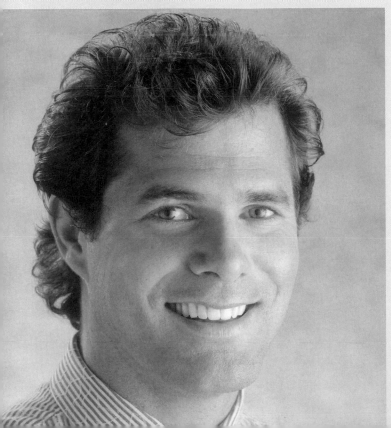

style no. 41

see page 35

style no. 42
see page 35

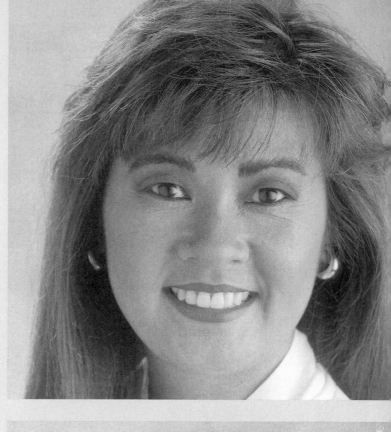

style no. 43
see page 35

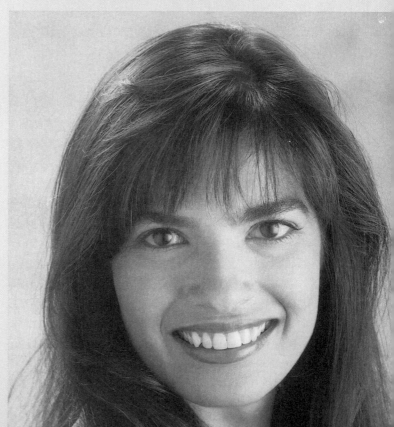

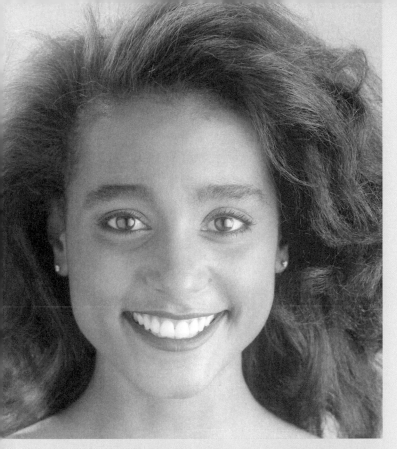

style no. 44
see page 35

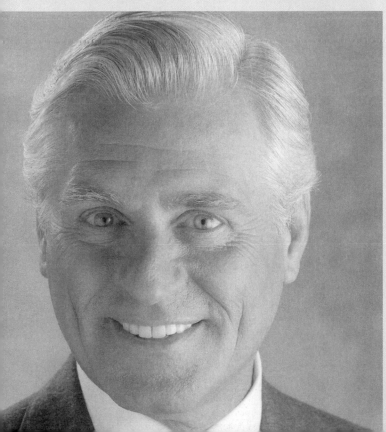

style no. 13
see page 32

style no. 46
see page 35

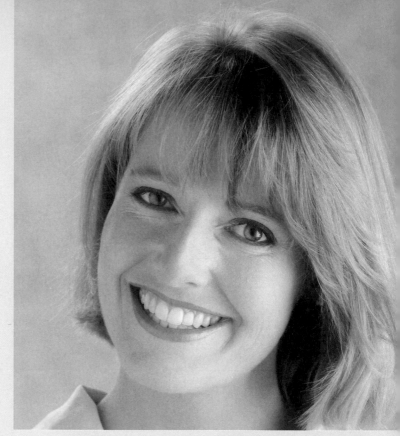

style no. 52
see page 36

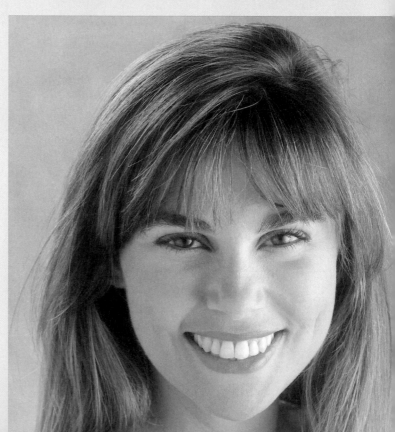

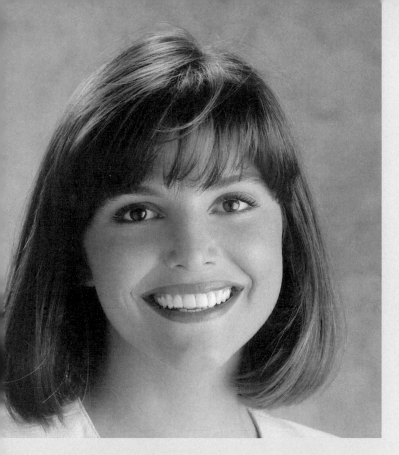

style no. 53
see page 36

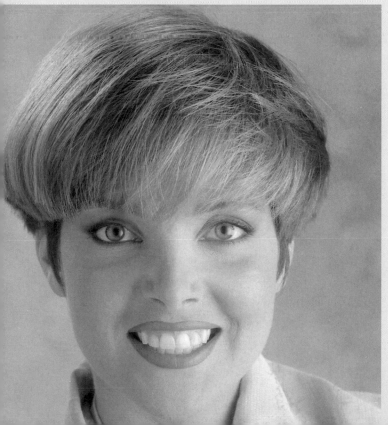

style no. 56
see page 36

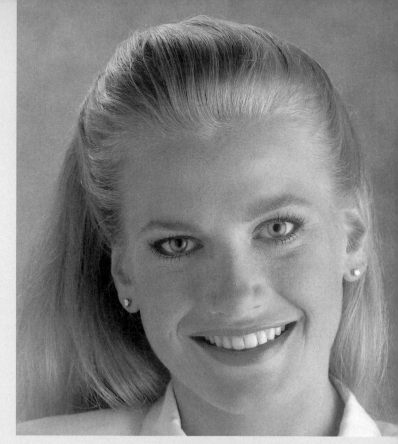

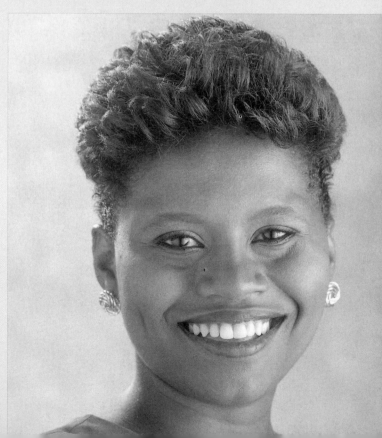

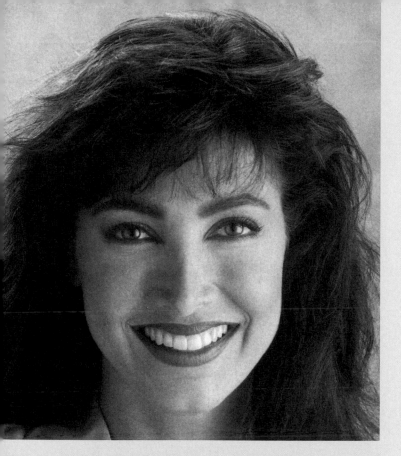

style no. 65
see page 37

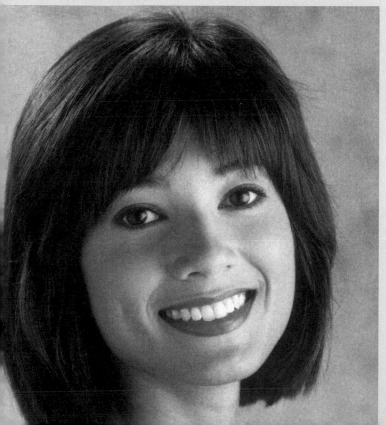

style no. 66
see page 37

Square Centrals
Square Laterals

	Central Incisor	Lateral Incisor	Canine	
style no. 11	square	square	square	
style no. 12	square	square	oval	
style no. 13	square	square	pointed	
style no. 14	square	square short	square	
style no. 15	square	square short	oval	
style no. 16	square	square short	pointed	

Square Centrals
Square Oval Laterals

	Central Incisor	Lateral Incisor	Canine	
style no. 21	square	square oval	square	
style no. 22	square	square oval	oval	
style no. 23	square	square oval	pointed	
style no. 24	square	square oval short	square	
style no. 25	square	square oval short	oval	
style no. 26	square	square oval short	pointed	

Square Centrals
Oval Laterals

	Central Incisor	Lateral Incisor	Canine	
style no. 31	square	oval	square	
style no. 32	square	oval	oval	
style no. 33	square	oval	pointed	
style no. 34	square	oval short	square	
style no. 35	square	oval short	oval	
style no. 36	square	oval short	pointed	

Square Oval Centrals
Square Oval Laterals

	Central Incisor	Lateral Incisor	Canine	
style no. 41	square oval	square oval	square	
style no. 42	square oval	square oval	oval	
style no. 43	square oval	square oval	pointed	
style no. 44	square oval	square oval short	square	
style no. 45	square oval	square oval short	oval	
style no. 46	square oval	square oval short	pointed	

Square Oval Centrals
Oval Laterals

	Central Incisor	Lateral Incisor	Canine	
style no. 51	square oval	oval	square	
style no. 52	square oval	oval	oval	
style no. 53	square oval	oval	pointed	
style no. 54	square oval	oval short	square	
style no. 55	square oval	oval short	oval	
style no. 56	square oval	oval short	pointed	

Oval Centrals
Oval Laterals

	Central Incisor	Lateral Incisor	Canine	
style no. 61	oval	oval	square	
style no. 62	oval	oval	oval	
style no. 63	oval	oval	pointed	
style no. 64	oval	oval short	square	
style no. 65	oval	oval short	oval	
style no. 66	oval	oval short	pointed	

imitation is the best form of flattery

3

smiles from the stars

CELEBRITY SCRAPBOOK OF SMILES

A great face, a killer body, talent, and of course a thousand-watt smile are some of the ingredients you need to make it in Hollywood. And I've had the privilege of helping some of Hollywood's biggest stars shine a little brighter.

Many people emulate stars: their taste in clothes, their hairstyles, their figures, and even their smiles. Every week someone comes into my office asking me to help her look like her favorite star. The smile most requested by my female patients is Halle Berry's, and other common requests are Julia Roberts, Cindy Crawford, and Claudia Schiffer. (It may just be a macho thing but my male patients don't ask for Brad Pitt's smile; in fact, they never name a celebrity.)

superstar smiles

This chapter discusses types of celebrity smiles and what these smiles suggest about personality, temperament, self-confidence, attitude, and sex appeal. They say imitation is the best form of flattery. We'll help you decide which celebrity smile might look best on you!

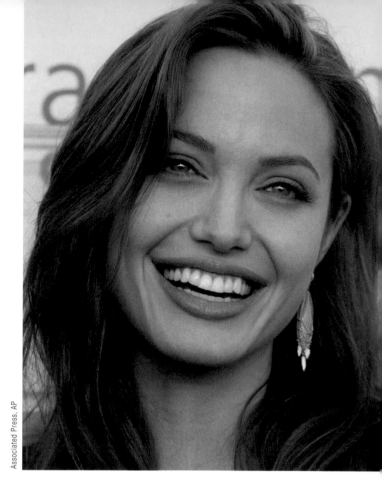

Associated Press, AP

ANGELINA JOLIE

Angelina Jolie's smile is one of the most seductive in Hollywood. It says, "Come close if you dare." It's mysterious as well. Her full, round lips complete the package. When she gives a great big smile, she looks like the friendly girl next door (if you live in Hollywood, that is).

Angelina's smile reveals a lot of teeth, even those in back. However, her mouth is a perfect example of a case where the teeth are less important than the lips. Her lips "make" her smile. The first thing that attracts you to her mouth is her full, voluptuous, seductive lips. They almost tease you to the point of curiosity until she reveals the teeth behind them, which don't let you down either.

She has big, beautiful, pearly whites that are as flawless as the rest of her. They have all the natural curves indicative of a Hollywood goddess and help make her probably one of the most kissable leading women today.

Angelina Jolie's smile is best suited for a younger woman with fuller lips, and would work well on any face except a round or square face.

OPRAH WINFREY

Oprah's smile projects confidence, power, and success.

Her teeth are slightly larger and more squarely shaped than usual. It's both a warm and a "don't mess with me" type of smile, depending on which look she wants to give.

Oprah's smile is her face's most dominant feature. It's what your eyes are drawn to, and she, in turn, draws you in with it. Oprah knows how to "work" her smile. Her dazzling white teeth make a beautiful contrast to her dark complexion.

Oprah's smile is appropriate for a woman with a big smile and a big personality.

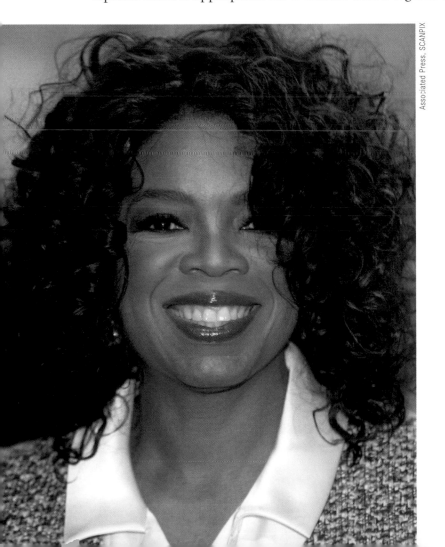

Associated Press, SCANPIX

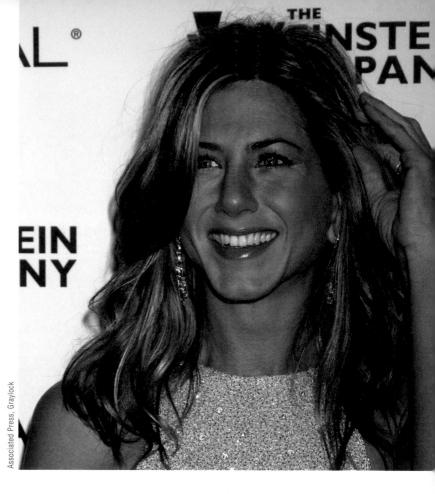

Associated Press, Graylock

JENNIFER ANISTON

With her clean, bright smile, Jennifer Aniston is the quintessential girl next door—an all-American beauty. As the world's most famous "friend," Jennifer made "the Rachel" hairstyles as popular as her show. But forget the hair! When I think of Jennifer's face, it's all about her smile. Jennifer Aniston's smile makes her look friendly and approachable. Her wide, happy smile gives her a healthy glow. Jennifer's smile is white but not shockingly white. Her sun-kissed, tan skin complements it well.

I think Jennifer's smile does what a smile is supposed to do. It illuminates her face. Her lips frame her teeth just right. Her teeth are feminine, rounded, and perfectly sized. You don't see gums or the bottom teeth. It's classic. It's symmetrical. It's pure. Her smile says the same thing as the *Friends* theme song: "I'll be there for you."

Jennifer Aniston's smile would work well on almost any woman, but works best on longer, more oval faces.

TYRA BANKS

Tyra Banks has a white, healthy, youthful smile that sparkles like her eyes and complements her rich complexion. Befitting her generous, warm personality, Tyra has a wide, revealing smile that exposes her proportionately sized teeth.

Her smile is always sweet, whether she's having a heart-to-heart conversation with one of the guests on her show or strutting down the runway in Victoria's Secret lingerie. Tyra's smile makes her approachable—she doesn't intimidate people the way some supermodels have a way of doing.

A Tyra Banks smile works best on an angular or long face.

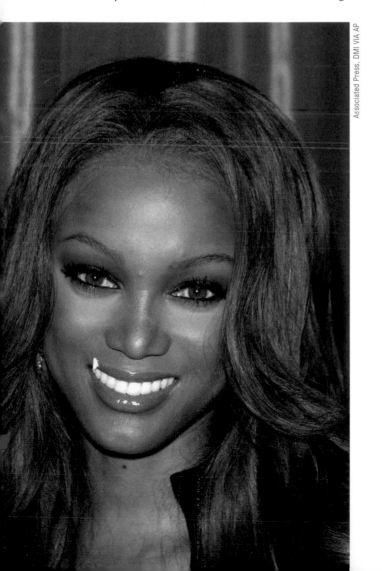

Associated Press, DMI VIA AP

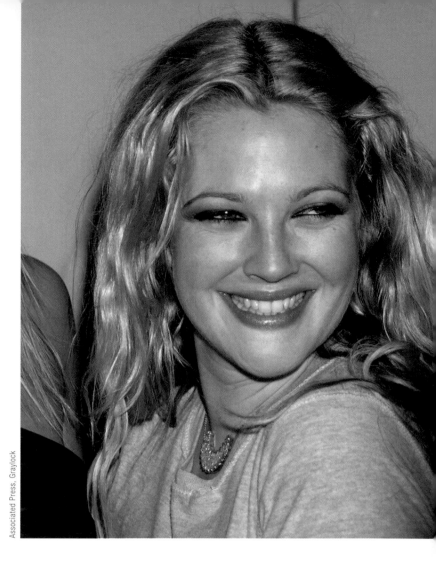

Associated Press, Graylock

DREW BARRYMORE

Drew Barrymore has a knowing smile, an "I've got a secret" kind of smile. The world fell in love with her as that little girl from *E.T.,* and although she's grown up to be a sexy, smart actor and powerful producer, she still has that sweet, winning smile.

Her smile is a little crooked in an endearing, adorable sort of way. Drew's smile is youthful, with smaller teeth that are not all the same length. She has a very natural shade of white. Drew doesn't need to prove anything to anyone in Hollywood. The former wild child is a survivor and a conqueror, and her smile matches her spirit.

Drew Barrymore's smile is for a woman with a youthful spirit and a round or square face.

MATT DAMON

Matt Damon could be Hilary Swank's brother (see page 60). They both share that big, toothy grin that makes them so approachable, likeable, and human. When Matt grins, his face lights up. With two front teeth that are longer than the others and a boyish face, he still looks like a teenager. But when he closes his mouth, he looks more mature.

Matt Damon's smile would be best suited for someone with a toothier grin and a round face shape.

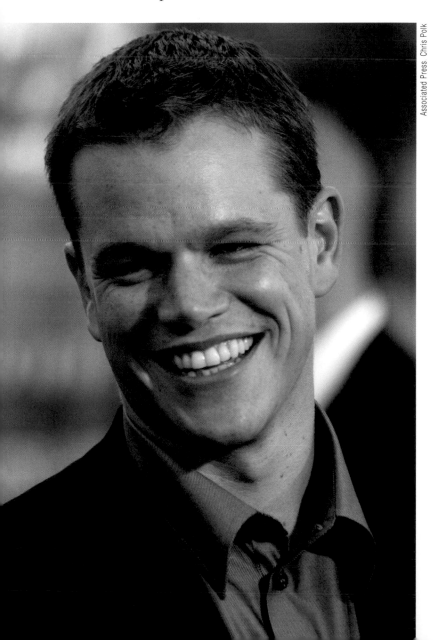

Associated Press, Chris Polk

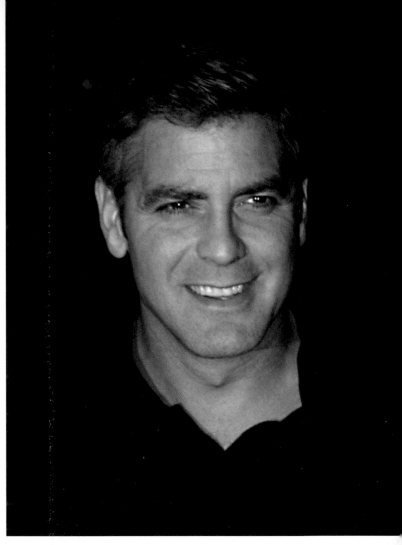

Associated Press, Arroyo

GEORGE CLOONEY

George Clooney has a debonair, devil-may-care smile. It's sophisticated and sophomoric at the same time. As a gifted actor and humanitarian, George is clearly an adult, but he jokes around like a kid—even when accepting his best supporting actor Oscar for *Syriana.*

With strong, even teeth, his smile is masculine and warm. George Clooney smiles with a twinkle in his eye, as if he's smiling at that special woman.

George Clooney's smile would be an asset to almost any man—it could help him look a little more masculine and a lot classier.

CINDY CRAWFORD

Cindy Crawford is the all-American classic beauty. Her long, cascading hair, flawless skin, full lips, and of course that famous mole frame her dazzling smile. Cindy's teeth are big, strong, symmetrical, and healthy looking. She was never a waif. This supermodel didn't fall into the skeletal chic category. She was always the epitome of healthy beauty.

Cindy truly looks like she eats an apple a day. Her smile says, "I am an American icon."

You don't need to be a supermodel to have a super smile like Cindy's. It would suit almost any woman and works well for round or square faces.

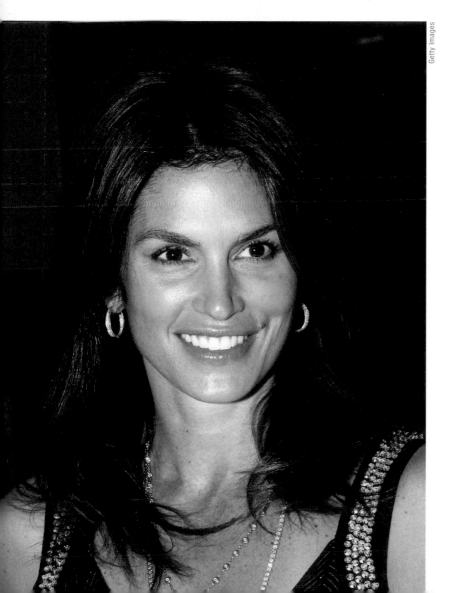

Getty Images

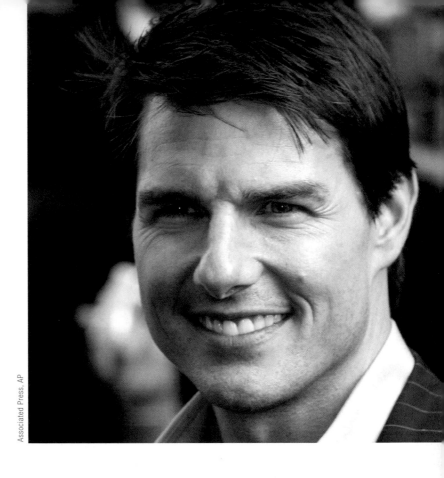

Associated Press, AP

TOM CRUISE

Tom Cruise's smile is a little mischievous. He seems to have gotten his mother Mary Lee's smile. If you've ever seen them together on the red carpet, you'll know what I mean.

Tom's teeth are a lot straighter now that he wore clear braces as an adult. His teeth are large and powerful, yet noticeably asymmetric. In fact, if you look closely, you will see that his midline (where the two upper front teeth meet, which should be the middle of your face) is nowhere near that mark. That imperfection makes him seem more human and more likeable. Even though he's one of the most photographed men in Hollywood and he could afford diamond teeth if he wanted, he still "keeps it real." He doesn't have that fake, picket fence smile. He looks like a guy who can get things done, a real player.

If you're a guy with more rugged features and not too much of a perfectionist, then Tom Cruise's smile might look good on you.

HALLE BERRY

Although Halle Berry is arguably one of the most beautiful women in the world, she doesn't have a traditionally feminine smile. Typically in women we see teeth that have more of an oval shape with rounder edges. And although Halle's smile is one of the most beautiful in Hollywood, it does not fit this mold.

Her super-white teeth are more squarely shaped than we are used to seeing on a woman. In her case, it doesn't detract from her femininity, but makes her even more appealing, stronger, sexier, and explosive.

In contrast to her delicate feminine features, her smile is a little bolder. Her smile says to me, "I may be beautiful but I have an edge."

Halle Berry's smile works best on oval or long faces.

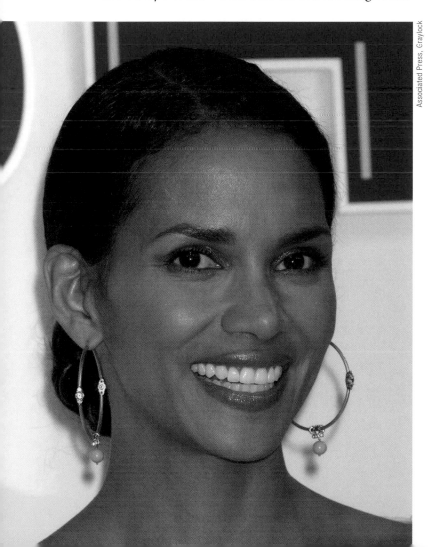

Associated Press, Graylock

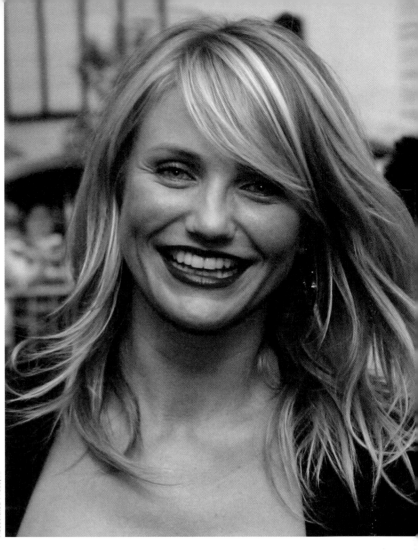

CAMERON DIAZ

Sexy and silly all at the same time, Cameron Diaz uses her smile to express her moods. Like Julia Roberts, Diaz has a great, wide, beautiful smile that you can fall right into.

Her upper lip line is perfect, falling just below the top of her well-proportioned front incisors. With her madcap "let's boogie" personality, it can be a zany smile, but when she wants to simmer, she can make it pouty and luscious. When she smiles, her smile says, "I'm groovy. I'm goofy. I'm gorgeous." Most importantly, Cameron's smile says she's happy in her own skin.

If you want to look like Cameron Diaz when you smile, you have to have a wide smile to start with, and ideally a long face.

LUCY LIU

Lucy Liu has a fresh, exotic smile that sings. Her teeth are clean, bright, and even. They are softly shaped and proportionate to her mouth. Her smile is a bright shade of white, which works nicely with her fair, porcelain complexion and dark, silky hair.

Lucy's smile says she's full of potential. But it's also a sassy smile. She's sweet but can be tough at the same time. Remember, this "angel" is a city girl who hails from Queens, New York. In *Kill Bill* her smile was as sharp as her sword.

A Lucy Liu smile would look best on a petite face with fine features that is either heart-shaped or long.

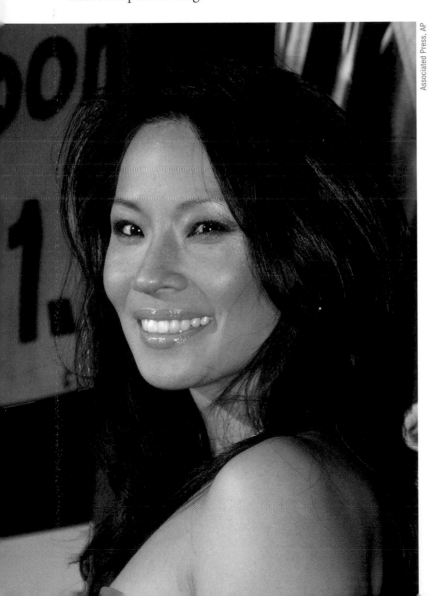

Associated Press, AP

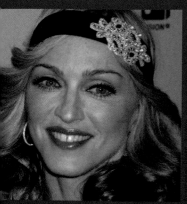
Madonna

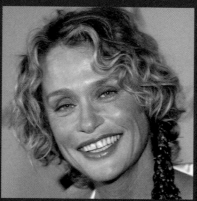
Lauren Hutton

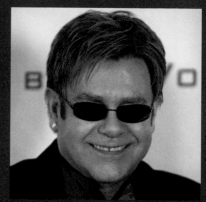
Elton John

FILLING IN THE GAP

What do Madonna, Lauren Hutton, and Elton John all have in common? Yes, they are all superstars, but that's not what I'm talking about. They all sport gaps in their upper front teeth.

Having a gap in your smile can convey several things about your personality. It can say, "I'm so good-looking that I don't care if my teeth aren't perfect." It can also say, "I'm not a perfectionist." A gap can add character to a smile. In fact, on several occasions I have actually had patients request a gap for just this reason.

People with gaps in their front teeth will experience one of three things and it's completely unpredictable. The gap will either stay the same, get bigger, or get smaller. In fact, in rare cases, predominantly in African-American women for some unknown reason, I have seen what was once a cute little gap in the teenage years grow to be so large that by age forty, you could put a whole tooth in the width of the gap.

There are no medical or health reasons to close a gap. If you don't want to be a part of the gapped-tooth clique, however, there is something you can do about it. You have several options. (You'll find more about all these procedures in Chapter 4.)

Bonding. If your teeth are healthy and it's a small gap of about three millimeters or less, a quick and conservative fix is to use tooth-colored bonding resin materials. Composite resin is used to close the gap by making the teeth on either side of the gap wider. Combined with contouring to even out the smile, bonding is an effective, quick way to fix gaps. It's also less expensive than crowning. The biggest drawback is that it's not very durable and the bonded pieces can be dislodged with flossing or hard foods.

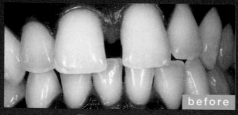
The gap between these two front teeth was closed with bonding.

Braces, retainer, Invisalign. An even more conservative solution would be braces, a retainer, or Invisalign (clear, removable, nearly invisible plastic or polymer "aligners"). All of these procedures are orthodontic and move the teeth into place without altering the physical structure of the teeth. That means no drilling! The disadvantage, of course, is that it's not a quick fix.

Veneers. For the most aesthetically pleasing and most durable instant repair, porcelain veneers can be placed on the teeth in two visits.

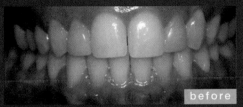
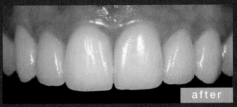
before / after

These teeth had a small gap and a lot of old bonding; porcelain veneers were used to create a perfect smile.

Crowns. In the same way a porcelain veneer is used, two crowns can be used to fill the gap, but a veneer is preferable because it requires much less tooth preparation, or filing down of the original tooth.

MOVIE STAR'S MAKEOVER

Brendan Fraser has the ultimate leading man smile: big, broad, and bold. In the film *Bedazzled* with Elizabeth Hurley, he plays several different characters from a high-strung, intense, nervous drug lord to a wishy-washy pushover kind of guy.

For the drug lord character, the makeup artists used a dental prosthetic that gave him the appearance of someone with a type A personality who takes out his aggression by grinding his teeth. They were flat and worn-down on the edges.

In contrast, when Brendan played the sappy, wimpy, and spineless character, the makeup artists used a dental prosthetic that gave him a less masculine-looking, rounder, and softer smile.

To a large degree, your smile typecasts you, and *Bedazzled* shows how even Hollywood bigwigs acknowledge that teeth help define different types of personalities and characters.

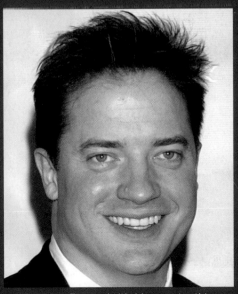
Brendan Fraser (with his own teeth).

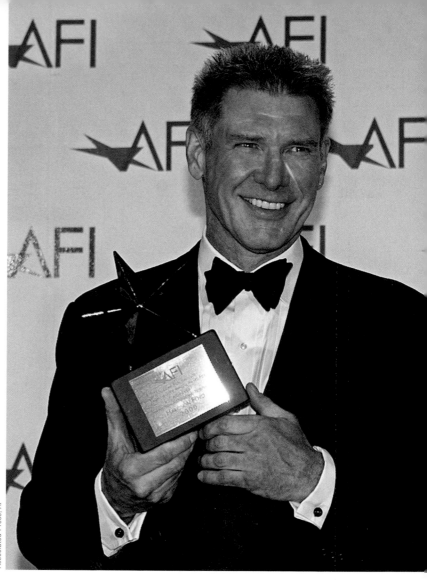

Associated Press, AP

HARRISON FORD

Harrison Ford is your classic, rugged Hollywood cowboy. His distinguished smile is decidedly masculine. He looks like the Marlboro man, but one who doesn't smoke. His smile is an age-appropriate shade of white, not "teenager white." His teeth are straight and strong. Their shape is also age-appropriate. His tooth line is straight across—a solid line.

His smile says, "I may be a guy's guy, but I know how to smooth-talk the ladies."

Harrison Ford's smile is perfect for a mature man with a younger man's spirit.

RICKY MARTIN

He may be living *la vida loca,* but Ricky Martin obviously has time to take care of his teeth! He has a broad smile with great teeth. Ricky also smiles with his eyes, which makes his smile seem more genuine.

His smile is more boyish than mature. It's a wide smile with teeth that are nicely shaped, white, and strong. Ricky's upper lip also falls nicely onto his teeth without showing gums. Ricky's smile explodes with a bang.

If you're a man with a wide smile, then Ricky's smile might be right for you.

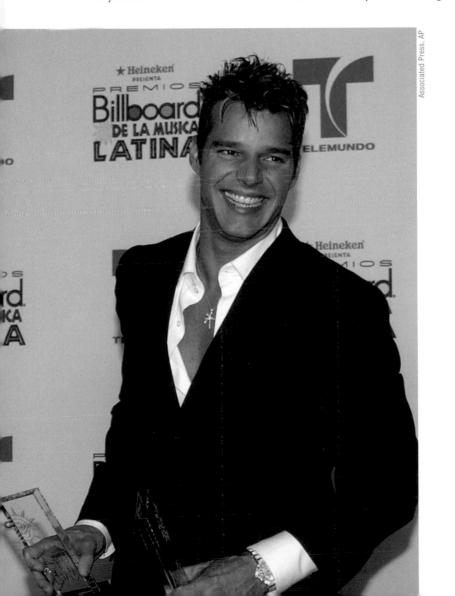

Associated Press, AP

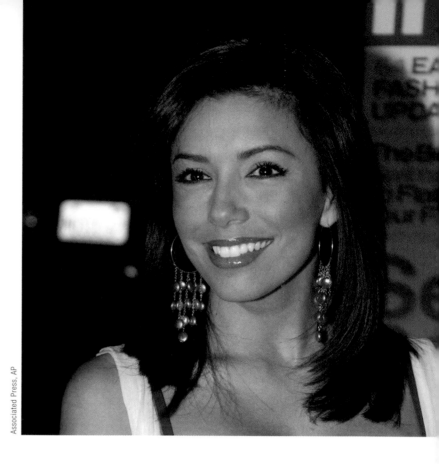

Associated Press, AP

EVA LONGORIA

There's nothing desperate about this desperate housewife, especially when she flashes you her sexy smile. When she plays the restless and conniving Gabrielle Solis on Wisteria Lane, Eva uses that pearly white, seductive smile to get her way.

Eva's smile is fresh and perky but with an edge. You see both her upper and lower teeth when she smiles. Her teeth are clean and very white, which works well with her darker skin tone.

Eva's smile is not textbook perfect, but it is perfect for Eva. Her teeth are not all even in length and are pretty big for such a petite woman. But Eva's full lips make the smile work—her plump lips frame her teeth proportionally.

Eva's smile would work well for a woman with fuller lips and an oval face.

KIRSTEN DUNST

Kirsten Dunst's smile is playful. And because it's not perfectly even, she's got a female version of that mischievous Tom Cruise thing going on. Her smile doesn't really flow. There are pronounced irregularities that show it's real and youthful.

Kirsten has smaller-sized teeth that are not perfectly shaped or aligned. Combined with her dimples and beautiful blue eyes, her smile declares, "I'm cute. I'm sweet. I'm lovable."

Kirsten Dunst's smile is ideally suited for young, sweet girls.

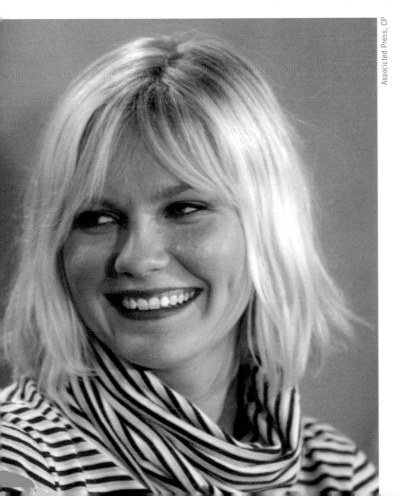

Associated Press, CP

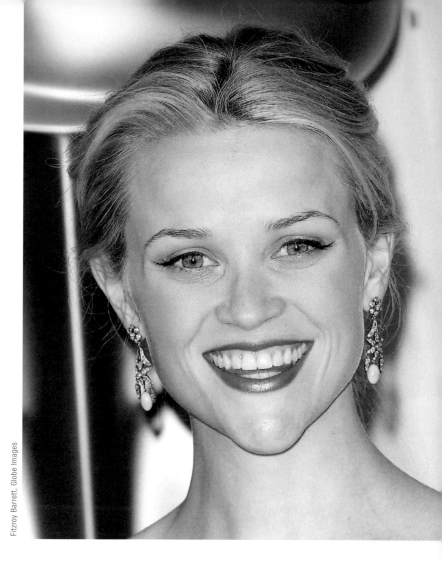

Fitzroy Barrett, Globe Images

REESE WITHERSPOON

Reese Witherspoon's teeth protrude slightly outward. She appears ambitious and aggressive but in a nonthreatening way, not unlike the over-achieving character Tracy Flick she played in the film *Election* or her Oscar-winning role as June Carter Cash in *Walk the Line.*

Reese's determined smile says, "I'll do whatever it takes to win and you won't even hate me when I beat you because I'm so sweet and adorable!" Her film company, after all, is called Type A Films.

Reese Witherspoon's smile is appropriate for a younger woman with teeth that protrude and would complement a long face.

JULIA ROBERTS

Julia Roberts's smile could light up all of Los Angeles. If the city tapped into the energy of her magnificent smile, power outages would be a thing of the past. Her smile is radiantly feminine, a prototype for the modern woman.

She shows all her teeth when she smiles. It's wide and carefree. Even though she's in her thirties, her smile appears younger with her even-sized teeth. There are no sharp angles. Her smile is soft, with no abrupt breaks. It flows from ear to ear with curves and fluidity.

When Julia Roberts turns her smile "off," you'd barely notice her, but when it's on, get your sunglasses out and enjoy the show.

If you have a wide smile and you want to be an even prettier "pretty woman," then Julia Roberts's smile could be your ticket. It could help a long or heart-shaped face appear broader.

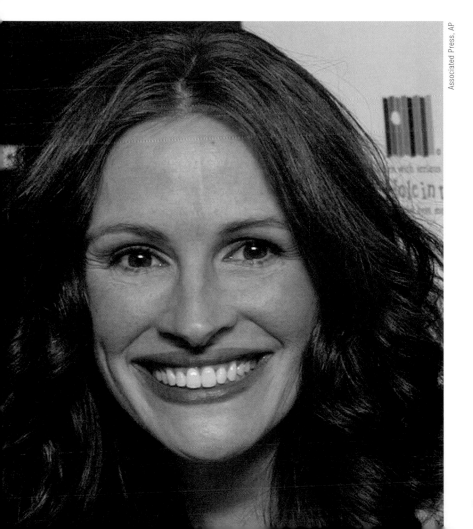

Associated Press, AP

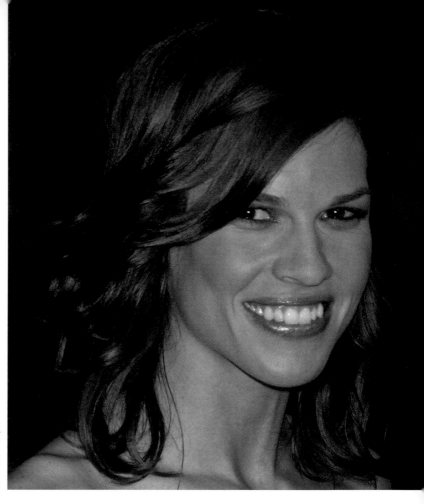

HILARY SWANK

Hilary Swank has one of the toothiest smiles in the business. It's very real, not perfect, but perfect for her. Her teeth are longer than what I might suggest for a smile makeover, but her unique smile lends itself well to the diverse, offbeat roles she takes on and gives her a distinctive look.

While a tad long, her teeth seem very healthy and strong. Her smile is ambitious, just like her. Remember, this was a girl who came to Hollywood with her mother as a teenager with nothing more than a dream. She's said that there were times when they slept in their car at night while she auditioned during the day. Her smile is fearless.

Hilary Swank's smile says, "I'm going for it because I've got nothing to lose."

If you have longer teeth, it's possible to duplicate Hilary Swank's unique smile. Her smile also could be used as a guide for shape in broad, square, or round faces.

DONALD TRUMP

Though you often see him with a scowl, this is a book about smiles, so I'm going to comment on those rare flashes when "The Donald" decides to show a little love and a big smile.

Trump actually has a very nice smile. The straight lines of his teeth are age-appropriate and very masculine.

You have to wonder why he doesn't reveal his smile more often. It's transformative. It flies in the face of his tough-as-nails persona. (I suspect he wants you to think he could fire you at any minute.) When he smiles, he's no longer "The Donald" you love to fear.

For a mature gentleman who is the boss, Donald Trump's smile could be a good investment and works well with almost any face shape. (Later in this book, I will share a personal story of how I "out-trumped" Trump.)

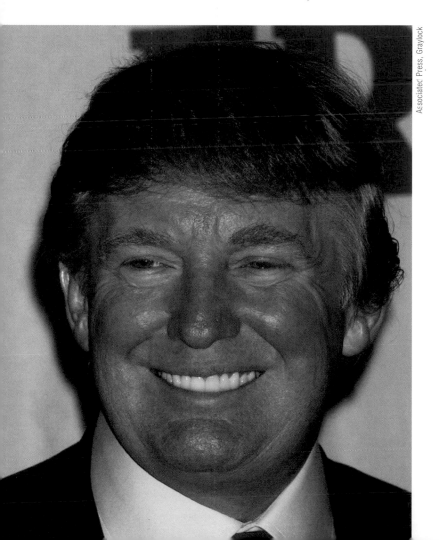

Associated Press, Graylock

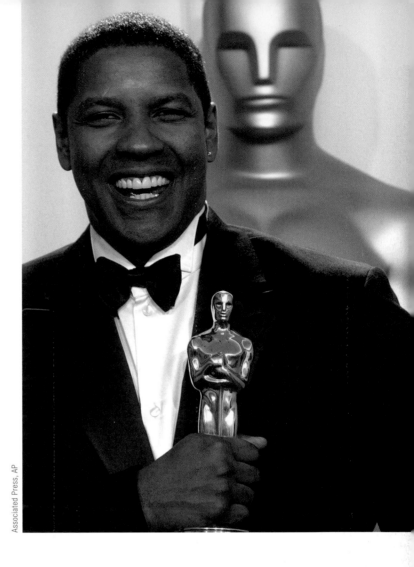

DENZEL WASHINGTON

Whether he is throwing punches as he did playing boxer Rubin "Hurricane" Carter or making speeches as slain civil rights leader Malcolm X, Denzel Washington commands attention, especially when he smiles. Denzel has straight, strong, prominent white teeth. His face is intelligent and intense when he smiles with his mouth closed, but his face instantly brightens up and becomes friendly and playful when he shows his teeth.

His smile is clean and happy when you see him freshly shaved. When Denzel is sporting facial hair, his smile softens and complements that tougher look. It's smooth and confident, just like the man who wears it.

Denzel's smile is for a man with a masculine face, strong features, and a big personality.

SNAP-ON SMILES

In our celebrity-obsessed culture, it is no great surprise that star-struck fans will do whatever it takes to emulate their screen idols.

Temporary veneers or snap-on smiles are one of the latest trends in dentistry. They're not cheap, either. They can run over a hundred dollars a tooth!

Temporary veneers use a special resin that's known for being flexible. A mold is taken of your existing teeth, and then the new veneers are glued onto the mold. Some are attached to your teeth with a temporary adhesive, while others snap into the nooks and crannies between your teeth. It's painless, of course, because it's attached simply by hand.

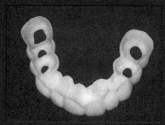
Snap-on smile.

The problem is that temporary veneers are not very strong and you usually can't eat or sleep with them.

I typically make them for actors and actresses as props in a commercial or movie when a certain smile is required. Up close, snap-ons usually are unnatural looking because they tend to be bulky and there's no real separation between the teeth—but if you happen to have small teeth with large spaces between them, the snap-on smile may look natural. Like most cosmetic trends, these temporary veneers are made popular by media hype.

I don't see a future for them in day-to-day life because they're like a Halloween costume. Their most beneficial use would be to allow you to preview a new smile and inspire you to have permanent veneers made, or to be used temporarily while you are saving money to correct a cosmetic dilemma.

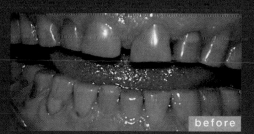
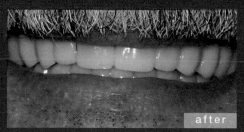
before
after

A snap-on smile conceals this patient's poorly spaced, discolored teeth.

how to construct your new smile

billion dollar smile manual

CREATING THE SMILE OF YOUR DREAMS

Did you ever buy a toy that required assembly? You wouldn't dream of putting it together without reading the directions first, right? You know what that toy can end up looking like if you don't follow instructions!

Think of this chapter as a Billion Dollar Smile instruction manual. It will educate you about your choices and help you navigate your way through the ever-expanding menu of dental options—and give you and your dentist a better idea how to construct your new smile.

This chapter will address the following questions:

> What procedure will work best for my problems?
> Am I a candidate for this particular procedure?
> What are the pros and cons of each procedure?
> What are the risks and benefits?
> How will the procedure feel?

Remember, the American Academy of Cosmetic Dentistry (www.aacd.com) recommends consumers consult with their dentist before undergoing any cosmetic dental treatment—this includes over-the-counter (OTC) products.

Now that you have determined what kind of smile you want, how do you get it? This chapter will identify all your cosmetic dental options.

Cosmetic dental treatment options include

> Whitening
> Contouring
> Bonding
> Veneers
> Crowns and permanent bridges
> Removable bridge (partial denture)
> Dentures (full)
> Implants
> Root canal
> Correcting gummy smiles with crown lengthening, lip repositioning, and orthognathic surgery
> Orthodontics

Note that although a root canal is not a cosmetic dental procedure, it is included in this chapter because it is often required before cosmetic procedures can be completed. At the end of the chapter, you'll also learn about the anesthetics that can make obtaining your Billion Dollar Smile as comfortable as possible.

whitening

Whitening is the most commonly prescribed cosmetic dental procedure in the world, and Chapter 5 explains it in more detail. You have many choices, depending on your budget and your lifestyle. You can have your teeth whitened an average of eight shades lighter in the dental office in less than an hour with an in-office whitening treatment, such as Discus Dental's product ZOOM! Or you can wear teeth-whitening trays during the day or overnight using take-home products from your dentist, such as Discus Dental's products Nite White and Day White. There are also whitening products available at the drugstore, but these are not as effective, and there are some risks (more on these in Chapter 5).

Whether you are a good candidate for teeth whitening depends on what type of dentistry you've already had done and what kind of teeth you have (teeth discolored from tetracycline or too much fluoride, for instance, may bleach unevenly). Keep in mind that only natural tooth structure will whiten, while veneers, crowns, and bonding remain their original color. So if you have a mix of natural teeth and restored teeth, after you whiten your teeth, you will need to have the synthetic parts replaced to match the new lighter color.

But I can't stress strongly enough—despite all the OTC products available at the drugstore—that whitening should be a dentist-supervised treatment. This isn't only for reasons of safety and effectiveness. Aesthetically, you should have some professional guidance.

contouring

Contouring, or shaping the teeth, is affordable and painless. Just a few minutes in your dentist's chair and you can completely alter the shape and personality of your smile. It is not unlike filing your nails: That's how painless it is for most people, because the nerve, also called the pulp, is buried in the middle of the tooth, and your dentist's tools are too far away from it to create any kind of sensation.

HOW IT WORKS

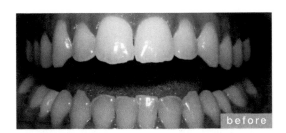
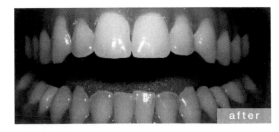

Contouring removed chips on the twenty-year-old female patient's upper front teeth, giving her smile a more youthful appearance.

A good candidate for contouring has healthy teeth that are uneven in appearance but with a fairly uniform U-shaped arch. Your arch is the shape you see when you bite into a sandwich. People with protruding front teeth, for example, do not have a uniform arch shape.

In contouring nothing is added to the tooth—only taken away. Basically, your dentist removes small areas of your tooth by sanding and shaping to resolve imperfections, like an artist might do to a sculpture. In the rare case where the procedure does feel uncomfortable, your dentist can give you local anesthesia, but I have had to do this only a few times in the last twenty years. Sometimes dentists combine contouring with bonding or a veneer or two to achieve a nice even smile. You can pick a smile by referring to the Smile Guide (see page 17) in Chapter 2 and by choosing teeth styles with your dentist.

Pros of contouring:	Cons of contouring:
> Quick	> Cannot be reversed
> Very minor sensation, like filing your nails	> Requires a uniform arch shape
> Inexpensive	
> Retains your natural tooth structure	

CONTOURING FOR COPYCATS

I once had a patient named Timothy whose best friend had just received a full set of porcelain veneers from me. Timothy was so impressed with his friend's new smile that he too decided he wanted all of his upper teeth veneered. Even though he was only in his mid-twenties, Timothy's teeth were yellow, crooked, and chipped. After a thorough examination, I explained to Timothy that I was confident that I could give him a flawless smile by just whitening his teeth and reshaping or contouring them.

Timothy was so insistent on getting porcelain veneers that he had already gone to the bank and withdrawn the same amount of money his friend had paid me. He handed me this big wad of cash, insisting I give him veneers. I kept explaining that, sometimes, less

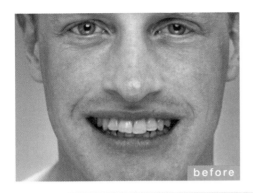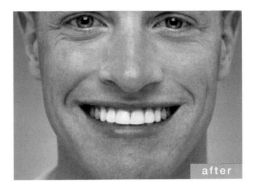

before after

Contouring and tooth whitening improved the appearance of Tim's uneven, dark teeth.

is best; sometimes, the best thing we can do for our smile is to keep the natural tooth structure and just enhance it. First work with what nature gave you.

I also explained that after whitening and reshaping, if he wasn't happy with the result we could always do more, but once you do porcelain veneers, you irreversibly alter a tooth and can never go back. Nothing dentistry can make will last as long as natural teeth that are healthy and strong, as Timothy's were.

After the shock that I wouldn't take his money wore off, he finally acquiesced, with the proviso that I would do porcelain veneers if he wasn't satisfied. As you can see in the photos, Timothy was more than satisfied with his new smile—and so was his accountant.

bonding

For more than half a century, dentists have been using a tooth-colored material called composite to bond, fill, or cosmetically enhance teeth. Composite is a mixture of resin, glass, and fillers that mimics the appearance and approximate strength of tooth structure. When you adhere this mixture to a tooth, the composite "bonds" to the tooth.

HOW IT WORKS

Bonding is often a viable option for repairing chipped, cracked, or disfigured front teeth and replacing silver amalgam on back teeth. An enamel-like material is applied to a tooth's surface, sculpted into shape, hardened by a laser or cure light, and then polished into your Billion Dollar Smile. When cosmetically enhancing your front teeth, anesthesia is not usually needed, and your new smile can often be completed in one visit.

Bonding can improve the appearance of upper or lower teeth by filling in cavities or imperfections, chips, uneven surfaces, and gaps. Bonding may be a good way to change the size, shape, and position of teeth. It is a lot less expensive and faster than orthodontic treatment, which can take years, and in some cases it is just as effective.

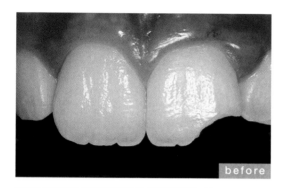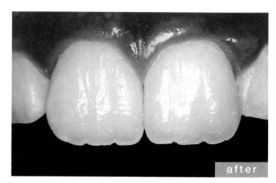

Bonding repaired this thirteen-year-old girl's chipped front tooth.

For slight rotations and small chips, bonding may last five to seven years. When more correction is needed, porcelain veneers are a stronger, more permanent alternative.

Because bonding isn't as strong as natural front teeth, you may have to be careful when biting into hard things like carrots and apples. Opening packages with your teeth and biting your nails can damage your natural teeth, but will annihilate bonding. Bonded fillings on back teeth are stronger than on front teeth, and you can typically chew whatever you want without a problem. You and your dentist will decide what works best for you.

And remember that bonding almost always will have to be replaced eventually—so if you plan on whitening your teeth, do it first, so the bonding can be matched to the new color.

At the first visit. Bonding the front teeth typically requires one appointment. The dentist may remove a very minor amount of tooth structure to maximize adhesion of the composite resin to the tooth, depending on the dentist's bonding technique. A tooth etching agent (a weak acid) is applied to the prepared tooth to create a microscopically porous matrix. This is coated with a clear adhesive resin, which flows into the pores and bonds the tooth-colored resin to the porous tooth structure. The dentist then contours the tooth-colored resin, which starts off in a dense putty-like consistency, to produce the desired appearance. Once this is satisfactorily accomplished, the dentist exposes the materials to a special laser or curing light to harden permanently.

Taking care of them. Teeth bonded or filled with composite resin should receive the same meticulous care as natural teeth. Regular brushing, flossing, tongue scraping, and professional preventive treatments are necessary to maintain proper oral health and appearance. To enhance the longevity and maintain the appearance of composite bonding, you should avoid excessive consumption of stain-producing foods and beverages (such as dark sodas, coffee, tea, and soy sauce) and the use of tobacco products. Habits such as nail-biting or using teeth to tear thread or other materials should also be avoided.

Pros of bonding:	Cons of bonding:
> Fast—usually one visit	> Breaks and stains more easily than porcelain options
> Looks natural	> Could end up with a mismatched smile if you bleach after bonding
> Very conservative (almost no tooth reduction required)	
> Relatively less expensive than more durable cosmetic options	

BONDING WITH CHELSEA

Chelsea, a beautiful twenty-something-year-old fitness model, came into my office with her boyfriend. He was having porcelain veneers done, so she wanted them done too. I suspect she didn't want her boyfriend's smile outshining her own! So I checked out her teeth and discovered they were healthy and in great shape, but she was unhappy with the chipped edges and misshaped smile line. Other than that, 85 percent of each tooth was in perfect condition.

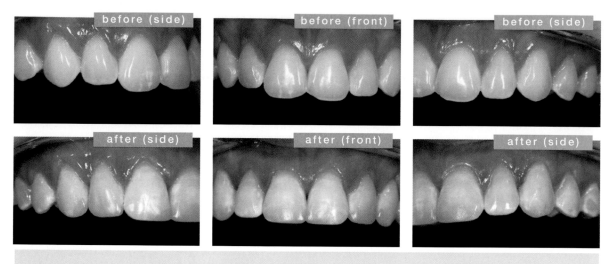

Bonding repaired Chelsea's chipped tooth edges and misshapen smile line.

Now, I could have used costlier veneers as I did with her boyfriend, but in her case it would have been overkill—and bonding usually looks more natural when you save a good part of the original tooth and only bond a portion of it. Our ultimate goal is always to look real, and nothing is as sure a bet for looking natural as maintaining your own tooth structure if at all possible. If all your tooth needs is enhancing at the edges or small changes, then bonding makes sense. Remember, you can always do more later, but you can't do less.

So I convinced Chelsea to give bonding a try and assured her that if she didn't like it, she could come back for porcelain veneers. It's been more than six years now, and she and I are still happy with the results.

veneers

If your dentist determines that you are a good candidate for veneers, they are probably the most aesthetically pleasing restorative option to shape up your smile. Veneers are ultra-thin, custom-made laminates that are permanently fixed directly to the teeth. They have become increasingly popular and are a great durable option for changing the size, shape, position, and color of teeth.

I placed my first veneer in 1986 on Mrs. McCarthy, who had been my neighbor since I was four years old, and it is still working perfectly. In fact, Danny Materdomini, the master ceramist who owns da Vinci dental studios, was at the chair side to help me, and since then I have used da Vinci veneers for all my cosmetic dentistry.

Veneers are used to close gaps, straighten teeth, replace worn edges, or resurface discolored teeth (usually brown, orange, or black) that for various reasons did not get white enough with the whitening procedures. The best candidates for all veneers are people whose teeth are healthy and free of decay and periodontal disease. However, cavities or tooth decay can often be repaired at the time of the veneer preparation.

If your front teeth are chipped or crooked or if you have a gap that is beyond what conventional bonding can cover, then veneers might be the best option. Unlike a crown, which covers the entire tooth, a veneer covers mainly the visible front part of the tooth and slightly wraps over the biting edge.

There are two types of veneers: porcelain (sometimes called laminates) and composite (resin) veneers.

HOW PORCELAIN VENEERS WORK

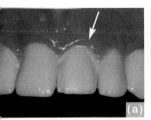 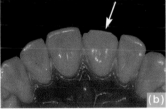 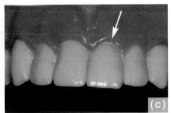 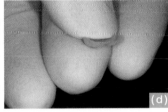

A tooth prepared for a porcelain veneer is shown on a model from (a) front and (b) back views; 0.5 to to 1 millimeter of enamel has been removed from the front and sides of the tooth. Notice that the back of the tooth (b) requires very little preparation because it will be almost entirely uncovered by the veneer. (c) The porcelain veneer is fitted on a model. (d) A porcelain veneer is about as thin as a fingernail.

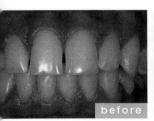 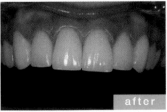 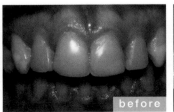 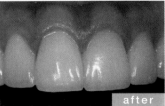

This patient had worn braces twice and still had spacing she did not like. Porcelain veneers closed the spaces and lightened the color of her teeth.

Old bonding was breaking off four front teeth, and the canines had mottled colors and an unpleasing shape. Porcelain veneers corrected the shape and color of the front six teeth.

Porcelain veneers are extremely thin tooth coverings made of durable dental ceramic. They cover only the visible part or front part of the tooth, hence the name "veneers."

At the first visit. First, you and your dentist select a smile style and color. I used to ask patients to bring in pictures from magazines, but now we can select a style from my book, *The Smile Guide.* For color, my preference is either to select a shade that matches the existing color or to bleach the rest of the teeth first and then match the new, whiter color. Sometimes patients want their new veneers slightly lighter than their existing color. (If you are going to whiten your teeth, it is important to do it *before* you get veneers, so the new color of the veneer can match the new color of the teeth.)

To make sure you know exactly what shape you are getting, I then use composite resin to make a "mock-up" of the selected smile style, directly on your teeth. Because anesthesia is usually not needed at this stage, we can see how the lips will naturally rest on the new smile. Once the shape is perfected, an impression is made to be used as a template for the temporaries and as a guide for the dental lab to copy.

Next, your dentist prepares your teeth by removing about 0.5 to 1 millimeter of enamel—about the thickness of your fingernail—from the front and sides so the veneer won't make the tooth look too big or bulky once it's attached. Your dentist makes an impression of the "prepared" teeth to be used as a guide to making your veneers in the dental laboratory.

Then your dentist puts temporaries on your teeth so you do not have to walk around with unsightly teeth. These are either pre-made or made in about fifteen to thirty minutes from the mock-up template, while you are in the chair. I like to make the temporaries look as close to the final veneers as possible. This is like a "trial smile," giving you a preview of the final product. Well-made temporaries may be indistinguishable from the final veneers for most people. In fact, I have had leading actors film big-budget Hollywood blockbusters wearing temporary crowns or veneers. And to my delight, even on the big screen, no one would know but the dentist.

If alterations are made to the original mock-up, a second model of the new shape is then sent to the lab as a guide to copy. So if you don't like your temporaries, don't keep it a secret—tell your dentist so they aren't copied for the permanent ones. While the temporaries look beautiful, they are not as strong as the final veneers, so you will have to restrict your diet to soft foods, and because they are all connected, flossing these teeth will be impossible. The final veneers, of course, will all be separate, individual teeth.

Most labs take one to two weeks to fabricate the final porcelain veneers. In special circumstances, some labs will do a "rush job" in one to three days, but this usually increases the fees.

At the second visit. When you return, your dentist places the final veneers on your teeth to check the fit, size, shape, and color—and to make sure you approve of your new smile. If adjustments are needed, they are made at this time. Then the veneers are permanently fixed or bonded to the teeth with resin cement.

I had four porcelain veneers made for my upper front teeth, and even though we did not change the shape or size much, it took me about a month to get used to the subtle size change to the point where they felt like my own teeth. This is a typical adjustment time for most people.

HOW COMPOSITE VENEERS WORK

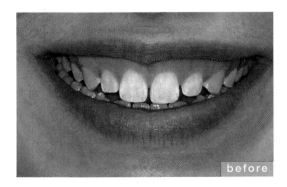
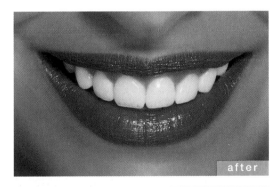

before after

Composite veneers were used to correct shape, color, and spacing.

Unlike porcelain veneers, which require two visits, composite (resin) veneers can usually be made in only one trip to the dentist. Another nice thing about composite veneers is that anesthesia isn't always needed and they are usually much less expensive than porcelain veneers.

Sometimes the patient's existing tooth must be prepared or shaped, as for porcelain veneers, but often no preparation is needed. In either case, your dentist applies a tooth-colored composite resin to your tooth and works his or her magic to sculpt the pliable composite resin material into beautiful, natural-looking teeth. A curing light is then shined on the pliable resin to permanently harden it. In the final step, your dentist smoothes out imperfections and polishes the resin so it blends in with your other teeth and looks natural.

Keep in mind that composite veneers are not as strong as porcelain veneers and are more susceptible to staining. As with porcelain veneers, it may take a few days to a few weeks to get used to the feeling of your new veneers because of the subtle shape difference.

Taking care of your veneers. You should maintain your veneers just like your regular teeth: with proper brushing, flossing, and regular dental checkups.

Veneers are beautiful but not indestructible, so you will have to take care of them. Avoid biting your nails, opening wrappers, or chewing on ice or your pencil. If you're a tooth grinder and do choose veneers to create your Billion Dollar Smile, try to curtail your grinding, and invest in a mouth guard to protect your smile while you sleep.

It typically takes as much pressure to break a porcelain veneer as it does a natural tooth. However, with proper care porcelain veneers can last many years or even a lifetime.

Pros of veneers:	Cons of veneers:
> More control over position, size, shape, texture, and color because they're custom-made for each tooth	> More expensive than other options, and porcelain veneers are more expensive than composite
> Fast, usually requiring just one or two visits; you may have your new smile in a few hours or within the week	> Usually require some of your teeth to be reduced
	> Irreversible when part of the tooth structure is removed
> Probably the most aesthetically pleasing and natural-looking restorations, and porcelain veneers are among the most durable restorations in dentistry	> Can chip or break (but it typically takes about as much force to break a porcelain veneer as it does a healthy natural tooth)
> Nearly as strong as a healthy natural tooth	> Tooth must be basically healthy and intact (if tooth is too damaged, you may require a crown instead)

Composite veneers are not as strong, and have a life expectancy of five to seven years. Keep in mind that veneers are almost always irreversible because the tooth is reshaped during the preparation process.

NO-TOOTH-PREPARATION PORCELAIN VENEERS

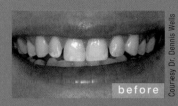
before
Courtesy Dr. Dennis Wells

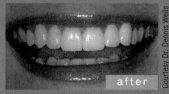
after
Courtesy Dr. Dennis Wells

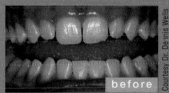
before
Courtesy Dr. Dennis Wells

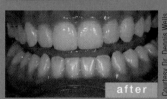
after
Courtesy Dr. Dennis Wells

Prepless veneers corrected the spacing in these two smiles.

Manufacturers claim that no-tooth-preparation porcelain veneers, or "prepless" veneers, can be a permanent cosmetic solution: a painless solution that can reshape, brighten, and whiten a smile.

The difference between these and regular veneers lies in the "no tooth preparation" part. So, unlike regular veneers, removing part of the existing tooth is not necessary. Sounds good, right?

The problem is that—unless you have very specific circumstances like lots of gaps, or teeth that slant in toward your tongue and need to be built outward—you usually end up with bulky, fake-looking teeth. With porcelain veneers you may remove as little as half a millimeter from the existing tooth and replace it with porcelain so it looks natural. Typically, unprepared veneers simply look too toothy. I'm not saying it should never be done, but case selection is critical for success.

There are very few cases where you get a nice, natural result, and again, that's generally on people who have teeth that need to be bulked out or made larger. So I usually tell patients, "No prep, no good." In my opinion, for a natural shape and size, you almost always have to remove some enamel and replace it with porcelain. The biggest problem with prepless veneers is that some dentists are overusing them and getting less than stellar results due to poor case selection. With proper case selection, however, the results can be beautiful. So just be cautious if you are considering this procedure!

HOW VENEERS HELPED TURN A "GOOFBALL" INTO A LEADING MAN

I had a celebrity patient on a hit sitcom who was being considered for a leading man in a feature film. His teeth were crooked and there were gaps and rotations. On a small television screen, his teeth didn't "read" so badly, but nevertheless he felt they made him look goofy (which was appropriate for his TV role).

In person and during the screen test for the feature film role, his goofy smile was even more obvious. The test went well and the studio loved him but told him he would only land the role if he got his teeth fixed. That smile just didn't mesh with the leading man-character he was being asked to play. This was a big break for the guy, so going to the dentist for that leading-man grin was a small price to pay for a chance to jump from being a TV star to a movie star.

Shooting was scheduled to begin within a few weeks, so time-consuming orthodontics weren't an option. It was veneers all the way for this hopeful Hollywood heavyweight. Together, we designed for him a leading man's smile: strong, straight, square, even, and masculine.

Up until that point he had played only comedic roles, but since we created his new smile, you've probably seen him woo his share of ladies on the big screen—and he has won his share of acting awards as well.

Even if you're not up for a leading role in a big-budget Hollywood movie, you have to be ready for your closeup every minute of your day, no matter what you do for a living. Your smile counts and you can't hide bad teeth when you want to flash a big, warm friendly smile.

crowns and permanent bridges

Crowns (also called caps), inlays, and onlays are dental restorations that are placed in or over a tooth when conservative restorations such as bonding aren't enough to restore form and function. Inlays and onlays are like a partial crown, usually made of porcelain. An inlay usually replaces a filling, while an onlay covers more tooth surface—it typically replaces a filling and covers one or more of the cusps of the tooth, and may cover the entire biting surface.

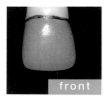

Porcelain-fused-to-metal crown.

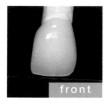
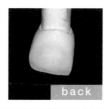

All-porcelain crown.

A bridge is a custom-made artificial tooth that fills in the gap where a tooth or teeth are missing, and attaches to the two teeth on either side. The replacement tooth or teeth are either attached to crowns placed on either side of the missing teeth, attached to the back of the adjacent teeth with wing-like appendages, or supported by dental implants.

Crowns and bridges can be made of tooth-colored material, metal, or a combination. Some metal-free crowns and bridges incorporate stress-bearing materials to make them stronger and wear longer.

HOW THEY WORK

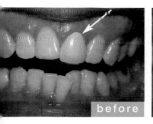
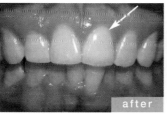
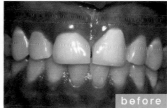
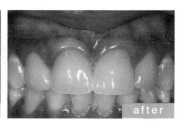

This old porcelain-fused-to-metal crown was replaced by a new all-porcelain crown. Notice how the dark line at the gumline of the crown disappears when there is no metal in the crown.

Before treatment, this patient had porcelain-fused-to-metal crowns on the two front teeth. Treatment included gum surgery, whitening, and the placement of all-porcelain crowns on the two central incisors (front teeth) and porcelain veneers on the lateral incisors. Notice how the colors of the crowns, the veneers, and the whitened teeth have all been matched so that they blend in perfectly.

Crowns address aesthetic needs, restore tooth function, and enhance the overall health of your mouth. Where back teeth have large broken-down fillings, a crown, inlay, or onlay can protect and preserve the remaining natural tooth. To enhance your smile, on the front teeth you can have an older porcelain-baked-over-metal crown replaced by a new metal-free, tooth-colored crown. All-porcelain crowns are similar to porcelain veneers except that more tooth structure is removed than with veneers, typically 1.5 to 2 millimeters in thickness all the way around the tooth, or more. And while veneers cover only the front of the tooth, a crown typically covers the entire tooth.

In one common type of bridge, the artificial replacement tooth, known as a pontic, is attached to two crowns, also called abutments. (The term "pontic" is derived from *pont,* Latin for bridge.) The crowns are cemented on the teeth on either side of the missing tooth, which support the permanent bridge.

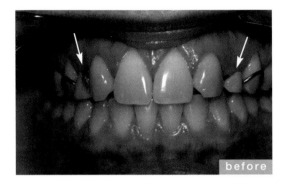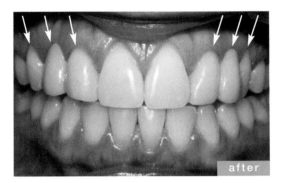

Before treatment, this patient was missing two teeth (indicated by arrows) and was wearing a removable bridge to fill the spaces. The patient was then fitted with two three-tooth permanent bridges (indicated by arrows); the natural teeth were also whitened.

A Maryland bridge is a relatively new type of permanent or fixed bridge that doesn't require crowns on the teeth on either side of the missing space. The dentist does a very minimal tooth preparation behind the tooth and bonds a "wing" type retainer to the back of the supporting teeth, which is then attached to the replacement tooth. Those wings can be made of either metal or a tooth-colored material. This type of bridge is usually more aesthetic and conservative because you don't have to remove as much tooth structure; it's also less expensive. Depending on the patient's bite, however, it may not be as strong as a conventional bridge.

At the first visit. With both crowns and bridges, the dentist shapes the teeth to provide stable support and precise fit of the final restoration. Following tooth preparation, impressions are taken of the teeth, and a replica of your mouth is created for the dental laboratory on a model to make the restoration. You and your dentist then carefully select the color, shape, and size of the crown or bridge. A temporary restoration is done to protect the prepared teeth and maintain the precise space left by the tooth until the new restoration is ready—and to keep you looking good.

At the second visit. When the crown or bridge is ready, the dentist removes the temporary restoration and tries on the crown or bridge to be sure it fits and that it meets your approval. Once the restoration is adjusted and approved, it is permanently secured with an adhesive bonding agent or cement.

Caring for your crowns and bridges. Crowns and bridges need the same meticulous care as natural teeth. Regular brushing, tongue scraping, flossing, and professional preventive treatments are required to maintain the appearance and health of supporting teeth and gums. Implant-supported crowns and bridges need additional attention: Ask your dentist about the selection of special flosses and cleaning instruments available to maintain hygiene, health, and appearance of these restorations.

Pros of crowns:	Cons of crowns:
> Can control size, shape, texture, and color (they are custom-made for each tooth) > On back teeth, restore aesthetics and function to broken, cracked, or filled teeth > Can be used on damaged or broken teeth	> More expensive than fillings > Involve more tooth reduction or preparation than veneers > Irreversible > Can chip or break, but are stronger than veneers
Pros of permanent bridges:	Cons of permanent bridges:
> Look, feel, and function more like natural teeth than removable bridges > Do not need to be removed from mouth for cleaning	> Cost more than removable bridges > Affect the adjacent teeth, to which they are attached > Can chip or break, and more teeth are involved than just a single tooth

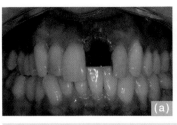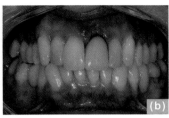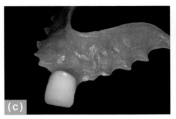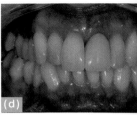

The removable flipper is usually just a short-term solution; it is often used after extractions, while a patient heals. (a) The tooth is extracted. (b) The removable flipper is inserted. (c) The flipper can be removed from the mouth. (d) Three weeks after surgery, the extraction site is still healing.

I have a patient who's a thirty-something famous rock-and-roll musician, a lead singer. When he was a kid, he fell off his bike and knocked out his front tooth. His family couldn't afford a permanent bridge, so he had one removable tooth made called a flipper. (Typically flippers are used short term and are often used while implants are healing.)

It looked okay since it replaced the missing tooth, but it was not ideal. He said it was really embarrassing kissing girls when the flipper would move. Once he had even spit his front tooth out while singing on stage!

So when he started making money he wanted a permanent bridge. I placed caps on the two teeth adjacent to the missing tooth and attached a permanent porcelain bridge.

The rock star kissed his flipper goodbye and millions of women hello!

removable bridges (partial dentures)

A removable bridge is also called a partial denture. You don't need to be a dentist to figure out that removable bridges need to be removed from the mouth for cleaning. They are less expensive than permanent bridges, which are usually are more stable and comfortable.

HOW THEY WORK

Some partial dentures are attached to implants, but most are attached to your permanent teeth with metal clasps. A Valplast partial denture is a metal-free removable bridge featuring clasps made of processed high-tech plastic that let your natural skin tone show through. The clasps wrap around the tooth at the gum line and should blend in with the natural color of the gums. You and your dentist will decide whether a partial denture with metal clasps or a Valplast partial denture will work best for you.

If the partial denture puts too much pressure on one area, your dentist can adjust it to make you feel more comfortable. With a new partial denture, an adjustment trial and error phase may be required. You need to start off slowly. In other words, eat soft foods initially, then work your way up to harder foods as your mouth acclimates to the prosthesis. I like to use the analogy that if you had an artificial leg, you would not run on the first day. Start off walking before you "run" to eating steak.

Most people remove their partial dentures after every meal for cleaning, and

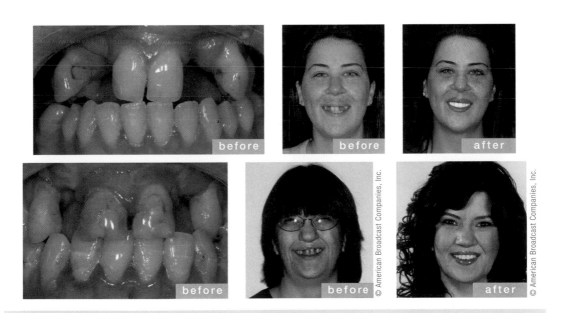

In patients with a cleft palate the teeth are usually too mobile for permanent bridges and there is not enough bone to support implants, so removable partial dentures are typically the best option. These two *Extreme Makeover* patients, Stacy Wiedenhoeft and Becky Powell, are sisters. Both received Valplast removable partial dentures to replace their missing front teeth, and porcelain veneers on the adjacent teeth to match.

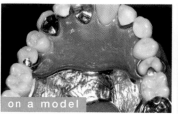
on a model

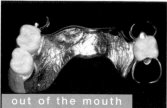
out of the mouth

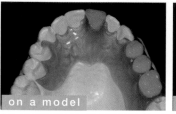
on a model

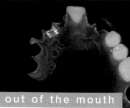
out of the mouth

Removable partial denture with resin and metal.

Valplast partial denture. Notice that the clasps are tissu colored to blend in.

although we suggest you sleep with them out, many patients wear full or partial dentures to sleep to avoid the embarrassment of being caught without a mouthful of teeth.

In fact, several patients who've been married for years tell me that their husbands have no idea that they wear dentures, because they never take them out in front of their spouses!

Keep in mind that your mouth changes as you age, so your partial denture may need to be adjusted, repaired, or relined along the way for better retention. Some of the material will be removed and it will be relined with new material to conform to the new shape of your mouth. (This is also true of dentures.)

For an option that does have a long list of cons, the removable partial denture is often incredibly effective. In situations where money is a factor or when implants aren't an option because of bone loss, removable partial dentures may be the best option. Also, if a patient doesn't want tooth structure removed to support a bridge, removable dentures are a viable choice.

I have a patient in his thirties who is fighting gum disease. As much as he would like to have a permanent bridge, the abutment teeth have so little bone support that they are not stable enough to hold a permanent bridge. I extracted the teeth that were hopeless and will continue to monitor the remaining teeth that have a hopeful prognosis. If the disease progresses over the years and he loses more teeth, we can add teeth to his removable partial denture or bridge.

At the first visit. Impressions and models are made of your mouth along with other measurements for the dental lab. You and your dentist then select a tooth shade (usually to match your other teeth) and tooth shape. Everything is sent to a dental lab.

At the second visit. The partial denture is usually returned to the dentist with the new teeth set in wax, so your dentist can "try it out." If everything fits properly, the partial denture is sent to the lab to be finished; if not, changes can be made in the wax.

At the third visit. Your finished partial denture is adjusted to fit comfortably. Additional appointments may be needed to "fine tune" the fit.

Taking care of your dentures. It's best to remove your partial denture after every meal for cleaning, and at night soak it in water with an effervescent denture cleaning tablet.

Pros of removable partial dentures:	Cons of removable partial dentures:
> Easier to repair than permanent bridges	> Can be less stable than fixed or nonremovable options
> Usually less expensive than permanent bridges	> Can break or be lost
> Can be used to replace teeth where there is not enough bone for implants	> Can be uncomfortable
> Can be used where there are not enough teeth to support a permanent bridge	> Usually have to be taken out at night for cleaning (but it is not mandatory)
	> Sometimes difficult to adapt to when speaking
	> May not be as aesthetic as other options

dentures

Dentures are usually viewed as a last resort if you can't afford implants or permanent or removable bridges. They are relatively inexpensive, the least expensive way to replace a mouthful of missing teeth.

But you should do everything you possibly can to avoid dentures. This is why the oral hygiene measures I keep harping about are so important, as are regular dental checkups. The sad truth is that in most cases, tooth loss does not have to happen.

With dentures, your chewing pressure can be reduced by over 75 percent. You also have to worry about dentures being dislodged during normal activities, such as eating. That's just no fun.

HOW THEY WORK

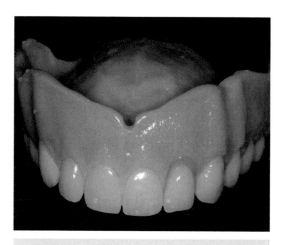

Full upper denture.

Most patients have total success with their upper dentures. They fit well, look great, and stay stable due to the support of the palate (the roof of your mouth). Outside of a few complaints of gagging or "not being able to taste food" (I'm not sure why this is an issue, but some people complain of it), upper dentures are easily tolerated.

Lower dentures are a different story. I've found that almost every denture-wearing patient hates them. I knew a wise old dentist who once suggested charging double for the upper denture and giving the lower one away for free!

The biggest problem is that they are not stable. Because your lower jaw moves up and down, there's constant motion, and you have no broad base support as you do with the upper denture on your palate—instead you just have a thin horseshoe-shaped ridge. And every time you swallow, your tongue lifts and moves the lower denture off this ridge.

Another problem is that over time most denture wearers lose bone on their ridges, and when this happens on the bottom, your denture has even less support. Denture adhesive can do an amazing job holding the upper denture in place even if bone is lost, because the palate makes a stable base. In the lower denture, however, adhesive may not work at all, because there's simply not enough surface area: When the ridge is gone, there's nothing for the denture to sit on. Implants, however, can slow bone loss—they apparently "stimulate" the bone, which in turn maintains bone mass—so implants under a denture may help in two ways: They can prevent bone loss and they can attach to the denture to help hold it in place.

At the first visit. The first step in getting dentures is to decide what you want them to look like. You can try to copy your original teeth before they started to break down, choose a picture from a magazine, or use the Smile Guide in Chapter 2. Next you need to select a shade. Most dentists will have special shade guides to choose from. The final aesthetic factor is selecting the gums. Dentures are made of resin, and typically darker-skinned people have darker gums too. Make sure you and your dentist select a gum shade that matches your pigmentation. Next, your dentist takes a series of impressions and dental records. Everything is sent to the lab to prepare for a wax try-in at the next visit.

HOW TO GET
THE MOST NATURAL-LOOKING DENTURES

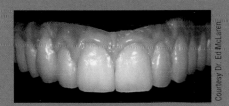

Courtesy Dr. Ed McLaren

Natural-looking full upper denture with blanched gums appearing around teeth.

For the most natural dentures, ask your dentist to give the lower front teeth very slight rotations or adjust the upper front teeth—or do both—so they are not all the exact same length. I like to make the two upper front teeth slightly longer than the others.

But the biggest tip is to request "blanched gum tissue." That means a slightly lighter resin is used at the gum line of each tooth to truly replicate nature. This adds a few hundred dollars to the cost, but it is money well spent.

At the second visit. First, your dentist has you try on your dentures mainly to check the bite and so you can approve how they look. The final teeth are set in wax at this appointment so changes can be made easily. Once they are approved, the dentures are sent to the lab to be finished.

At the third visit. Usually one week later, the final dentures are delivered to your dentist. After you've approved the aesthetics, the key to dentures is fit. If they fit well, they will be comfortable, more functional, and less likely to fall out. They will also look better and more natural.

If your dentures don't fit well or cause discomfort, you must tell your dentist. Don't settle for discomfort. Dentures should never be uncomfortable and a good dentist will completely share this belief. (But keep in mind there is a break-in period of one to two weeks while you adjust to the feel of your dentures.)

Taking care of your dentures. It's best to sleep without dentures to give your mouth a "rest." After you've removed them, rinse your mouth to clean it. Brush your dentures gently to remove any food debris, then soak them in water with an effervescent denture cleaning tablet. Most dentists recommend then brushing them again, as you would your natural teeth. Clean all surfaces, including where the denture contacts your gums. If stains build up, ask about having them cleaned at your dentist's office.

Pros of dentures:	Cons of dentures:
> No worry about brushing and flossing throughout the day, because you take them out at night for cleaning > No more toothaches	> Loss of your natural teeth > Can be uncomfortable, and some people even gag on them > Can look fake > Are removable > May affect taste and limit what you can eat > Bottom denture may not adhere well > If your bone continues to diminish, can become increasingly difficult to wear over time, because there's nothing for the denture to hold onto

A DENTURE DO

I once had a patient named Martha who wanted and desperately needed a smile makeover.

Martha knew her teeth looked terrible, but she was completely unaware that they were practically falling out of her mouth. They had been gradually getting looser and looser over the years but she wasn't aware of the extent of her periodontal (gum and bone) disease. When I told her she'd be losing all of her teeth, she broke down in tears.

Problem was, she had so much bone loss because of the periodontal disease that we had to extract all her teeth. Because Martha didn't have enough bone to anchor implants and didn't have any teeth to do a bridge, we had no other choice but to make a denture.

Even though I say dentures should be a last resort, these looked amazing. In this case, dentures were Martha's only hope for a normal smile. She now has the beautiful smile she had dreamed about.

implants

They're not just for breasts anymore! Dental implants replace lost or missing teeth. Implants are precision-crafted pieces of biocompatible metal (your body will not normally reject this material) that are surgically placed beneath the gums to fuse to the jawbone. They are in effect artificial tooth roots, to which a new tooth is attached.

In 1952 a Swedish orthopedic surgeon named Per-Ingvar Branemark, while studying bone healing in rabbits, discovered that a titanium rod had actually fused to the bone. He named this process osseointegration, and began researching using titanium screws as anchors for missing teeth. After years of research, the implant was born.

HOW THEY WORK

Today implants are a common procedure. Implants are used to replace one or more missing teeth, to support nonremovable permanent bridges for multiple teeth, or to better support a full or partial denture with clasps or retention bars (for photos of an implant-supported retention bar, see page 92). Because they also help maintain bone, they can help prevent additional tooth loss and a sunken facial appearance.

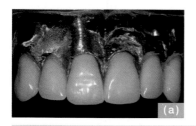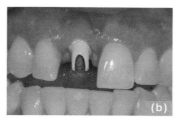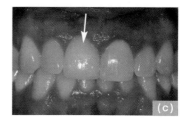

(a) A resin model shows how an implant is placed in the upper jaw. (b) An integrated implant with a white abutment was placed in this patient's jaw so that a natural, translucent, all-porcelain crown could be used without dark metal showing through. (c) A porcelain crown was then cemented on the implant. The patient also had tooth recontouring and orthodontic treatment.

Three separate pieces are involved: the implant (which fuses to your bone), an abutment that screws on the implant, and a crown that is cemented or screwed on the abutment.

Once the implant, usually made from titanium, is surgically placed in the bone, it takes four to six months for it to become integrated into the jaw. A life-like ceramic porcelain tooth restoration is then matched to the original tooth color and attached to the implant abutment. These feel more natural than conventional replacement bridges or dentures.

To be a candidate for implants, you must be healthy and have healthy gums and enough bone to support the implants. If you do not have adequate bone, an additional surgical procedure can often be used to augment your bone so implants can be done at a later date.

Implants can be very expensive and usually involve one or more surgeries over a few months. Although it may take up to six months for the bone to grow around the implant and firmly hold it in place, "immediate load" implants have recently become popular. Immediate load implants are just that. If you have excellent dense bone quality, there is sometimes enough support for the implant to bear the weight of light chewing and a tooth replacement right away. (An X-ray and CT scan are necessary to determine if bone density is adequate for this procedure.) It is so exciting when a patient who has been wearing dentures for many years can come into my office and after one long appointment walk out with implanted permanent teeth!

Usually implants can be placed with the patient awake; however, general anesthesia can be used upon request. If necessary, pain medications and in some cases antibiotics are prescribed.

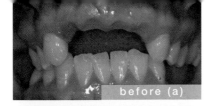

before (a)

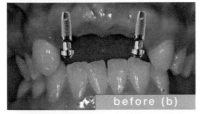

before (b)

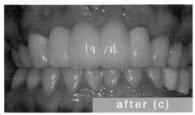

after (c)

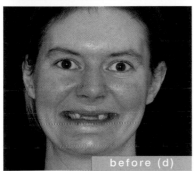

before (d)

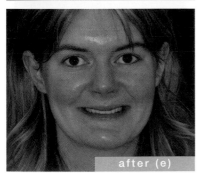

after (e)

(a) This patient was missing four front teeth. (b) A graphic illustration shows the placement of the two implants. (c) After the implants were placed, a four-tooth bridge was permanently placed, dramatically improving the patient's smile (d–e).

At the first visit. Your dentist will likely take an X-ray to determine the appropriate site for implant placement; some may prescribe CT scans as well. Impressions are taken of the mouth to aid in proper implant placement and possibly for the dental laboratory to use in creating a customized temporary restoration.

At the second visit. The dentist, usually an oral surgeon or periodontist, places the implants in the desired position in the bone. Once the metal implant is secure, the gum tissue is sutured back over the implant. The implant is left undisturbed for three to six months to allow it to "osseointegrate" or mesh with the bone. If the implant is in a visible area of the mouth, the patient may wear a temporary prosthesis during the healing period (a flipper or temporary cemented bridge). Dentures may be relined with soft liners so they can be comfortably worn during the healing process. (With immediate load implants, the implant is put into the bone and the tooth is attached right away, but not everyone is a candidate for this procedure.)

At the next visit. Once the implant has completely integrated with the bone, at the next visit the dentist may need to make an incision to expose the top of the implant. Sometimes the implant is not buried under the gum; it depends on its placement and how much gum tissue is in that area. Then a small metal post called an abutment is attached to the implant. The dentist then creates the permanent tooth replacement, which is placed on the abutment.

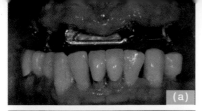

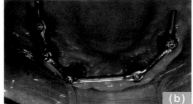

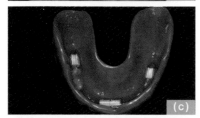

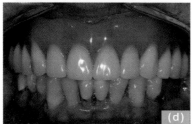

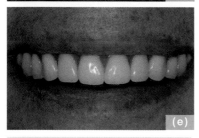

The implant-supported bar for Shannon's clip-on denture is shown from (a) front and (b) top views. (c) The full denture has yellow clips that fit on the bar. Note that without the clip and bar retention system, an upper denture would not be U-shaped and would have to cover the entire roof of the mouth for support (compare the photo of the full denture on page 86). (d) The upper denture clips on to the implanted support bar for a natural smile (e).

Taking care of your implant. Like natural teeth, implant restorations require regular daily oral care and professional dental hygiene appointments. People vary in their overall health, oral hygiene habits, and anatomical requirements, so each case is unique. But, provided they are well cared for and the patient remains healthy, dental implants can last indefinitely.

HOW IMPLANTS GAVE A "DESPERATE" HOUSEWIFE BACK HER SMILE

Shannon was a middle-aged housewife who saw her smile deteriorate over the years through neglect and bad genes.

She started getting cavities and experienced bone loss. So many of her upper teeth were extracted because of decay and bone loss that she ended up needing to wear a full upper denture, which she hated. Shannon said it made her feel old like her grandmother. She also complained that it gave her a "caved in" look when she took the denture out. But her biggest complaint was that because she had a strong gag reflex, she was actually gagging on it a lot of the time.

There wasn't enough bone to replace all her upper teeth with implants, so I placed as many implants as possible and made a solid bar that clipped into a thin, sleek, and incredibly stable denture. This clip-on denture gave her the benefit of a full set of teeth, just like a regular full upper denture. However, the clip-on denture was much more secure and did not cover her entire palate like a regular denture.

Often as people age, the bone underneath missing teeth melts away, making implant placement impossible without invasive bone augmentation. So if you are considering implants, time is of the essence.

Shannon was glad she did it. Not only does she love her new smile, she's not gagging anymore and she's able to eat whatever she wants again. And she looks ten years younger.

Pros of implants:	Cons of implants:
> Most similar to natural teeth > Can be placed without altering or grinding down adjacent teeth > May prevent shrinkage of the jawbone caused by tooth loss	> Not for everyone because of the bone structure required > Not recommended for smokers because smoking disrupts the healing process (the implant won't integrate into the bone) > Problematic for insulin-dependent diabetics, who tend to lose implants because of healing problems > Time-consuming and require more dental visits than alternative procedures > More expensive than other options—but in my experience, nearly 100 percent of patients agree that they are worth it

root canals

When the nerve of a tooth dies or becomes infected because of decay, trauma, or unknown factors, a root canal must be done. This even *sounds* painful—but it doesn't have to be. Root canals, also called endodontic treatment, can save a tooth that would otherwise have to be extracted because of infection or disease. A root canal procedure removes the diseased tooth's pulp (the nerve) and then seals off the root from the surrounding tissue so there will no longer be an infection. You can often save a severely decayed and even infected tooth through a root canal.

HOW THEY WORK

A root canal involves the removal of the tooth's pulp, that tissue thread of nerves in the center of the tooth that is in effect the blood supply of the tooth. After the nerve is removed, your dentist will seal off the space left from surrounding tissue.

It is usually best to save a tooth because natural teeth are almost always stronger and more aesthetic than artificial teeth. If a tooth is removed and not replaced, the neighboring teeth may shift in the mouth, ending up crooked or bunched up, and cause even more problems. And a crowded mouth is more susceptible to gum disease and cavities because it's harder to keep all those teeth properly cleaned and to floss between crowded teeth.

So how do you end up with a root canal anyway? What exactly goes wrong? When your pulp—the soft tissue inside the tooth containing blood vessels, nerves, and connective tissue—becomes diseased, it starts to die. This can be because of deep decay, trauma, or sometimes for no apparent reason. If the diseased pulp is not removed, the tissue dies and rots, leaking toxins into the tissue around that damaged tooth. Left untreated, the area becomes infected and an abscess can form. Lots of pain and swelling could result.

Ninety-five percent of the time, a root canal is a win-win situation—no pain, all gain. A restored tooth can last a lifetime with proper oral hygiene. However, even under the most ideal circumstances, 5 percent of all root canal treatments will not last for life. Failures occur when the tooth becomes reinfected or cracks. When a root canal fails, the tooth must be extracted, and can be replaced by either an implant or a bridge.

At the first visit. Usually a root canal takes more than one visit and can be done by your regular dentist or an endodontist, a root canal specialist. First, local anesthesia is administered. The tooth is isolated with a rubber dam and then an opening is made through the top or back of the tooth directly into the pulp chamber.

Then the pulp (the nerve) is removed from the pulp chamber and the root canals. The canal is cleaned in preparation for filling. Medication is usually put into the pulp chamber and root canal to eliminate bacteria. At the end of the first appointment or at a second appointment (if it was not possible to finish the treatment all in one appointment), the root canal is filled with a biocompatible material, usually gutta-percha, and then sealed. To fight infection, your dentist may also prescribe oral antibiotics.

At the final visit. At your regular dentist's office, the tooth is "restored" by a crown, veneer, or a filling made of tooth-colored composite resin or porcelain.

One last note: Once a tooth needs a root canal, you have only two choices: root canal or extraction. It will never heal on its own, and usually the longer you wait, the worse the situation becomes. The infection will grow, making the whole ordeal more painful, and it could spread to adjacent teeth. *The bottom line:* Don't wait—see the dentist when you have a toothache or swelling.

There are no pros and cons at the end of this section, because if you need a root canal, you really don't have a choice! You either have the root canal or have the tooth extracted, because the infection, if untreated, can be life-threatening.

how to treat the gummy smile

If your smile is too "gummy," with too much gum showing when you smile, there are several surgical techniques that can correct the problem.

Ideally the "perfect" position for your upper lip when you're smiling is to just rest at the level where your gums meet your two front teeth (as shown in the "after" photos in this section). Often a combination of two or more procedures is used to obtain the optimal results. Your dentist and either a plastic surgeon, an oral surgeon, or a periodontist (gum and supporting tooth structure specialist) will do the surgery. Surgical choices include crown lengthening, lip repositioning, and orthognathic surgery.

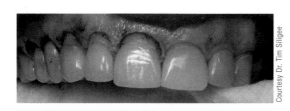

Courtesy Dr. Tim Siligee

In crown lengthening, gum tissue is removed (left side of photo) to lengthen the teeth and reduce a gummy smile.

CROWN LENGTHENING

This surgical procedure removes and recontours the gum tissue. An oral surgeon, periodontist (gum specialist), or cosmetic dentist removes some of the gum tissue

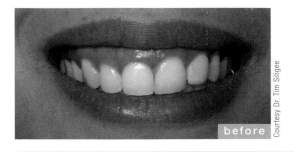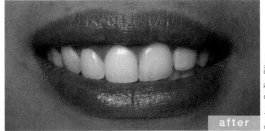

before

after

Crown lengthening evened out this patient's gum line.

above the tooth, making the teeth longer. This is done surgically, under local anesthesia, with a laser, scalpel, or electrosurge (this is an electrocauterizing instrument).

Crown lengthening is ideal when there is excess gum tissue covering short teeth. Once the gum tissue is removed, the teeth will appear longer. In some cases exposed root will now be showing, so porcelain veneers will be needed to aesthetically enhance the teeth. (In the cases pictured on this page, the roots remained covered so there was no need for porcelain veneers.) If you already have porcelain veneers, you will most likely need a new set to cover the root surface.

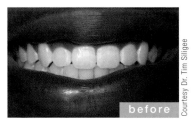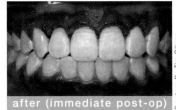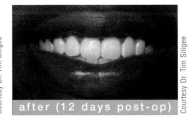

before

after (immediate post-op)

after (12 days post-op)

Excess gum tissue covered this patient's short teeth. Laser crown lengthening improved the patient's smile.

As scary as this procedure may sound, it is relatively fast and easy, and patients tolerate it well and heal quickly. If only a small amount of gum tissue is removed, healing is instantaneous; if some of the bone around the teeth is removed, full recovery may take one to two weeks. This procedure is done in one appointment and usually takes one to two hours, and can be done under local anesthesia. If you're really apprehensive, however, talk to your dentist about considering general anesthesia.

Pros of crown lengthening:	Cons of crown lengthening:
> Quick > Easy > Inexpensive > Predictable results > Usually no recovery time	> Limited success in some cases > May expose root of the tooth and thus require veneers

LIP REPOSITIONING

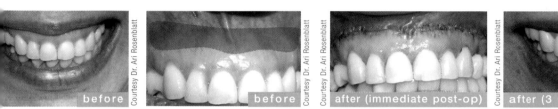
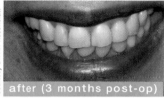

before — before — after (immediate post-op) — after (3 months post-op)

Courtesy Dr. Ari Rosenblatt

This patient needed lip repositioning to correct a gummy smile. The shaded area indicates the tissue that needed to be removed to tack the lip down. Note that after the surgery was fully healed, the upper lip was ideally positioned to touch the area where the tooth meets the gumline.

This simple yet dramatic procedure was brought to national attention when we began using it on *Extreme Makeover* to help correct gummy smiles. In the past the only ways to help were crown lengthening, which may not completely correct the problem, and orthognathic surgery, which is quite invasive. Although lip repositioning is not a new technique, it was mainly being done by plastic surgeons, and because it is not a highly profitable procedure, it fell by the wayside. I personally prefer to have a periodontist do this because they operate in the mouth all day long.

Today, lip repositioning is almost always used in conjunction with crown lengthening, but it can also work as a stand-alone procedure. It will generally correct a problem if the lip needs to be repositioned ten millimeters or less.

In this procedure a small portion of the tissue on the inside of your upper lip is removed and the lip is sutured to the gums. This limits the muscles that raise your lip

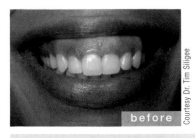 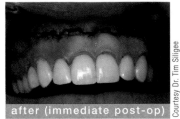 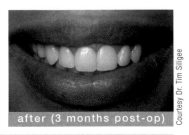

before | after (immediate post-op) | after (3 months post-op)

Courtesy Dr. Tim Siligee

Lip repositioning and crown lengthening corrected this patient's gummy smile.

from showing too much gum tissue. The procedure will not change the appearance of your face, but will stop your lip from rising up too high when you smile.

It is usually done under local anesthesia, and the procedure lasts around forty-five minutes. Often there is some swelling, particularly the first few days, but usually it is barely noticeable after a week and completely gone in two weeks.

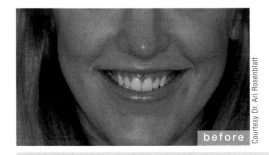 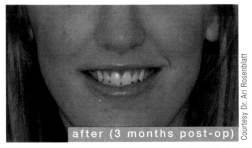

before | after (3 months post-op)

Courtesy Dr. Ari Rosenblatt

After lip repositioning, patients note a significant improvement in their gummy smiles without other changes to their faces.

Pros of lip repositioning:	Cons of lip repositioning:
> Fast	> The surgeon can only move the lip a limited amount
> Easy	> May need to be used in conjunction with crown lengthening to solve the problem
> Dramatic results	
> Quick recovery	
> Relatively inexpensive	
> Can alleviate the need for orthognathic surgery, with changes that can be just as dramatic	

ORTHOGNATHIC SURGERY

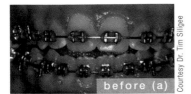

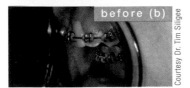

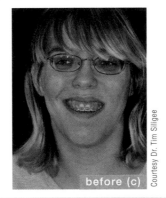

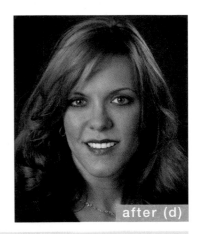

This patient had several skeletal problems that required orthognathic surgery. (a) Notice that even when she bit on her back teeth, her front teeth did not close. (b) She had a severe overbite, as shown in this side view. (c) She also had a gummy smile. (d) Orthognathic surgery, lip repositioning, crown lengthening, contouring, and ZOOM! whitening corrected her smile.

In the past this radical surgery, which involves movement of the jawbones, was the only effective way to get rid of a gummy smile. The upper jaw is detached and a section of bone is removed to shorten the length so that the lip will cover the gums. Usually a patient will have orthodontic treatment to position the teeth in as ideal a position as possible before this treatment. The surgery can take anywhere from a few hours to as long as eight hours. Once the oral surgeon is finished with the surgery, braces are used to wire the mouth closed for a period of about one month while the bone fuses. Healing can take as long as several months in some cases. This surgery can also be used to move the lower jaw forward or back to correct a patient's profile.

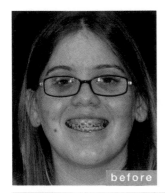

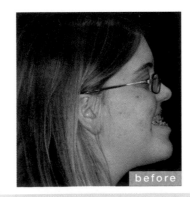

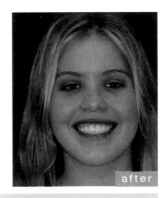

Orthognathic surgery can be used to move a patient's lower jaw back to improve the profile. This patient had orthognathic surgery, lip repositioning, six upper porcelain veneers, and ZOOM! whitening to correct her smile.

Pros of orthognathic surgery:	Cons of orthognathic surgery:
> Effective in severe cases that cannot be corrected by other means	> Very expensive > Jaw needs to be wired shut after surgery > Difficult to avoid losing weight with jaw wired shut > Difficult and lengthy healing period

YOU CAN CHANGE THE COLOR OF YOUR GUMS!

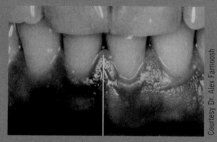

To illustrate the effectiveness of gum bleaching, half of this patient's mouth was bleached. On the left side of the white line is the gum that hasn't been treated. On the right side is the gum that has been treated and has healed for two weeks. Note the dramatic difference in color and appearance.

You may have the most beautiful, even, white teeth in the world—but if your gums are discolored or have dark patches, you aren't going to have a Billion Dollar Smile.

Even though common perception may be to the contrary, dark gums are not a health issue, but they can affect how your smile looks. Until the 1990s, not much could be done about dark gums. Now it is possible, however, to have your gums bleached in a relatively new procedure, using a series of chemicals that act somewhat like a chemical peel for skin. It's a simple technique, done in your dentist's office, and produces only minimal discomfort. There's no recovery time involved—you will be able to eat and speak normally right away.

Ask your dentist about this procedure, and for more information see www.dralexfarnoosh.com.

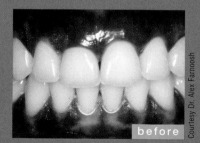
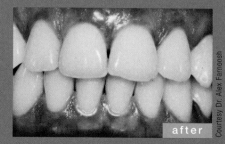

Gum bleaching corrected the color of this patient's gums. Note that this patient also had crown lengthening to reshape the gums for symmetry.

FROM GUMBY TO GORGEOUS

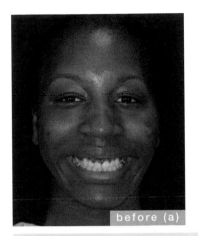 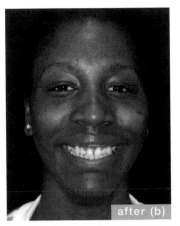 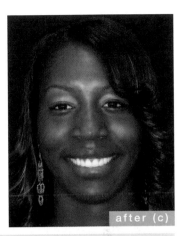

(a) Deidra required several procedures to correct her gummy smile. (b) First she had lip repositioning and crown lengthening. (c) After the surgery healed, her teeth were whitened and six porcelain veneers were placed.

A young woman named Deidra was teased mercilessly and called Gumby. She needed it all: lip repositioning, gum repositioning, whitening, and porcelain veneers for that Billion Dollar Smile.

As you can see from the photographs, her smile was gummy with too much gum tissue on her upper front teeth. (In addition the gums were a dark pigment that she did not like.) Because this gum tissue had to be eliminated with crown lengthening, we did not consider gum bleaching. However, when she smiled, you still saw too much gum tissue. So the periodontist and I did crown lengthening with a lip repositioning procedure to tack her upper lip down to prevent it from lifting and exposing a gummy smile.

After these procedures, when Deidra smiled, the teeth were perfectly framed in her mouth. The bottom portion of her upper lip just touched the area where her upper front teeth meet at the gum line. And the icing on the cake? We whitened her teeth with ZOOM! in-office whitening treatment and placed six porcelain veneers on her upper front six teeth.

Remember, a beautiful smile isn't just about teeth. It's a package deal, involving your gums and lips as well.

orthodontics

Braces aren't just for kids anymore. Remember when Tom Cruise had a slightly plastic-looking smile? I don't mean plastic, like superficial; I mean the clear braces he wore to help straighten his teeth.

Orthodontic treatment straightens crooked teeth and corrects what is known as mal-occlusions, or bad bites. Your dentist usually will refer you to an orthodontist if you or your child is a candidate for braces. Pressure on the teeth from the braces, retainers, or trays that are pushing the teeth toward the correct position causes bone in the path to dissolve. Where there is negative pressure (in the area that follows the moving tooth) bone growth is stimulated. In essence your teeth slowly move through bone, and bone grows to support your teeth in their new position.

The four main reasons to get orthodontic treatment are

1. Crowded teeth
2. Crooked teeth
3. Poorly aligned teeth
4. Poor upper and lower jaw alignment

Orthodontic patients usually begin full treatment around age twelve to fourteen—but orthodontics can be for everyone. It all depends on your dental situation and the type of smile you're trying to create. Children as young as five years old can receive orthodontic treatment to help their bones grow in properly, and certainly no one is ever too old for orthodontic treatment. The length of treatment can vary anywhere from several months for minor corrections to a year for moderate cases, and two or more years for more severe cases.

When it comes to full orthodontic treatment, you have four options: standard metal braces; clear braces; lingual or concealed braces (applied from the inside); or Invisalign, the nearly invisible plastic or polymer "aligners" mentioned earlier.

After your treatment, you will have to wear a retainer to keep that fabulous-looking smile looking fabulous. There are three options: a removable plastic device with one wire in

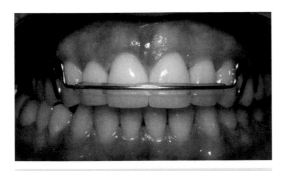

After orthodontics a retainer must be worn at night to prevent the teeth from relapsing to their earlier positions. This one has a metal wire, but other types may be wireless.

the front, a "permanent" retainer with a wire or fiber bonded to the back of your lower front teeth, or a clear plastic device that looks very much like the Invisalign trays. Normally, for the first few months you must wear a retainer full-time. Then, under the direction of your orthodontist, you can cut back to wearing it at night and every other day, and then just at night. Some people can eventually wear the retainer only occasionally at night, while some people will have to wear it forever. Without a retainer, your teeth can fall right back into the places where they were before you began treatment. How's that for incentive to wear your retainer?

CONVENTIONAL BRACES (METAL AND CLEAR)

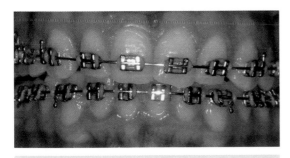

Metal braces.

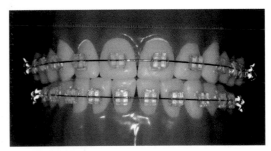

Clear braces.

Metal braces are less expensive than other types. Unfortunately, in addition to being unsightly, traditional metal braces make your teeth nearly impossible to clean properly. Brushing and flossing become a real challenge when you can't get in there to do your job. You know what that can lead to: tooth decay and gum disease.

You can opt for clear braces, with tooth-colored brackets made of ceramic rather than metal. For both metal and clear braces, a bracket is cemented to each tooth and a wire threads through the brackets. Clear braces are more aesthetic than metal ones, but also more fragile and more expensive.

Your first visit. Before you get your braces, your orthodontist makes a series of records of your teeth, including X-rays and models, and evaluates them carefully.

Your subsequent visits. When you return to the office, the orthodontist applies the braces. Additional appointments are then scheduled so the orthodontist can tighten and adjust the braces at regular intervals.

Pros of conventional braces:	Cons of conventional braces:
> Least expensive > May be a slightly faster treatment than lingual (concealed) braces or Invisalign > Moves teeth better in severe cases	> Not pleasing to look at (although clear braces are less obvious) > Difficult to clean teeth > Uncomfortable > Not removable > Many foods are on the "not allowed" list > Wires can break

LINGUAL (CONCEALED) BRACES

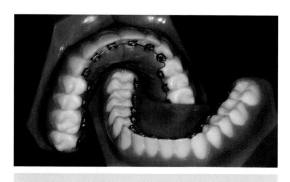

With lingual (concealed) braces, the brackets are placed on the inside of the teeth.

Lingual braces are placed on the inside, or tongue side, of the teeth, so they are concealed from view. Usually the concealed braces are conventional metal braces. Some people choose lingual braces on their top teeth, and conventional clear braces on the bottom teeth, because bottom teeth don't show as much as top teeth.

Your first visit. As with conventional braces, your orthodontist takes a mold of your teeth. Brackets will be positioned from this, and put in a plastic applicator.

Your second visit. Your orthodontist puts cement on the back of each bracket, presses them into place, and breaks off the applicator. Your orthodontist then puts an arch wire on the back of your teeth, which is threaded through the brackets. Because the arch wire is shaped in the position your teeth should be in, it helps pull your teeth into place.

Pros of lingual braces:	Cons of lingual braces:
> Most aesthetic of all braces	> Most expensive type of braces
	> May require longer treatment
	> Difficult to clean
	> Speaking may be more difficult
	> May not work for some types of alignment problems (consult your dentist)

INVISALIGN

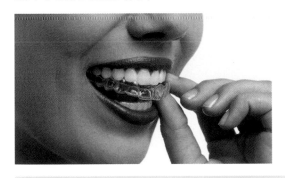 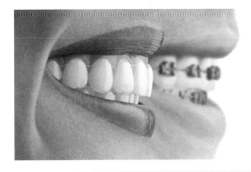

Invisalign tray being inserted (left) and in the mouth (right). The tray is almost invisible, especially compared to conventional metal braces.

Invisalign—nearly invisible, custom-made plastic or polymer trays—is changing how many adults are dealing with orthodontic options. For the most part, Invisalign is fast and easy.

These trays are a virtually painless way to straighten teeth. In addition to being nearly invisible, they are removable, which is especially good for eating and for brushing and flossing your teeth. (In fact, you change them every two weeks.) That's a great thing because many people with braces end up with perpetual gum inflammation because they simply cannot brush or floss properly.

According to the Invisalign company, about 80 percent of adults who require orthodontic treatment can use this product. You can even put whitener in the trays and kill two birds with one stone, resulting in teeth that are both straight and white.

Unfortunately, not everybody is a candidate for Invisalign. The 20 percent of adults who cannot use Invisalign usually have teeth that require more force than Invisalign can provide to rotate or move their teeth in a certain direction. And children can't use Invisalign until all their permanent teeth are in.

SMILE LIFT

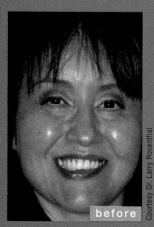
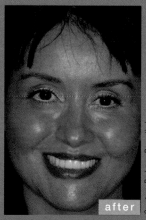

before

after

Courtesy Dr. Larry Rosenthal

A smile lift improved this patient's smile. Her teeth, especially the back teeth behind the canines, were built up and made a little thicker, creating a broader smile and a more youthful appearance.

A smile lift is like a face-lift for your smile.

If you feel your upper lip is too flat and your smile is too narrow, you can "pump it up" a bit with veneers or crowns. The upper teeth are built up and made thicker so the upper lip protrudes more, producing a boader smile. The overall effect is similar to that of collagen injections.

This procedure only works on certain people. It's not just an answer for thin lips. You have to look at the whole face. That's why it's important to go to a smile artist. The only way to know if you are a good candidate for this procedure is to have your dentist make a "trial smile." He or she can make temporary crowns or veneers using removable tooth-colored resin, or use a snap-on smile, to give you a preview of what the permanent ones will look like. This way you can take it for a test drive and see if the smile lift you're hoping for isn't too much or too little for your face.

Your first visit. Your dentist takes an impression of your teeth, and Invisalign uses this with the dentist's specific directions to make a series of customized teeth aligners.

At your second visit. You are given your first three sets of aligners, and if needed, attachments (small, nearly invisible tooth-colored bumps that are bonded to the tooth to aid in rotation of the tooth) are applied to the tooth as well. Plus, if teeth are crowded, a series of sanding strips may be used to make the teeth narrower.

Your subsequent visits. You get your next three sets of aligners, and any tooth adjustments are also made. Typically, you are seen every six weeks and given three new sets of aligners (each aligner is to be worn for two weeks at a time). The average treatment time is less than twelve months.

Pros of Invisalign:	Cons of Invisalign:
> Almost undetectable	> Cannot be used when teeth need more force to move or rotate them
> Easy to remove for eating and brushing and flossing	> May be slightly longer treatment
> Can whiten teeth at the same time	> Must have your permanent teeth in (cannot be used for children)
> No interference in teeth cleaning (just remove the tray)	> May be more expensive than other types of braces in some cases
> Your last tray can be used as your retainer	

anesthetics and sedation: so you don't feel a thing

Of course, you want your beautiful new smile to be as pain free and stress free as possible. Fortunately, your dentist has a number of anesthetics and sedatives available to make you comfortable.

LIDOCAINE FOR NUMBING

There isn't a dentist in America that uses novocaine anymore. Actually, the most common injectable anesthetic that we use to numb patients is called lidocaine. Novocaine was a very early form of anesthesia, but the general public doesn't realize it was replaced by lidocaine. I've never even seen novocaine!

Typically, dentists use nitrous oxide (laughing gas) to relax you, and put topical anesthesia on your gums so they can administer the injection of lidocaine most comfortably. Once you get the injection and you're numb, you're fine. It's getting the injection that's the hardest part.

LAUGHING GAS MAKES DENTISTRY A LAUGHING MATTER

The not-so-funny name for laughing gas is nitrous oxide. If you took chemistry in high school you can probably figure out what nitrous oxide consists of: It's a compound of nitrogen and oxygen. Dentists use it often as a sedative because it's effective and safe and has few side effects. And it makes you laugh! But more importantly, it heightens your threshold for pain.

With nitrous oxide you're not a total zombie, so you can answer your dentist's questions during the procedure. Laughing gas is typically used for all kinds of oral surgeries and tooth restorations and is usually used in conjunction with injectable anesthesia.

Laughing gas doesn't numb you—it just temporarily makes you feel really, really drunk. Even if you feel something, you just don't care.

For some patients that are incredibly anxious about being in the dentist's chair, we might use it for procedures that for most people do not cause discomfort. For example, we sometimes use it for patients who gag during mouth X-rays.

Laughing gas is dissipated through your system a minute or two after removing the nitrous oxide nosepiece. You should feel back to normal immediately. The only downside is that occasionally patients complain of headaches, during or after treatment. On rare occasions, it causes some patients to vomit.

The numbing effect of a typical injection of lidocaine lasts anywhere from one to four hours, depending on your metabolism. It's used to deaden the sensory perception of your teeth. That means it numbs you so we can do our job without hearing you complain about it!

The most dangerous side effect, although very rare, is an allergy to the medication. If you are allergic, the first time you receive lidocaine you'd usually experience a rash, swelling, or difficulty breathing, but the second time you'd typically have a much stronger reaction, which could be life-threatening. Fortunately, there are several types of anesthetics, and if you've had any sensitivity to lidocaine, you should see an allergist to determine a safe alternative.

Another common side effect is called tachycardia, an increase in your pulse rate. It's like that feeling you get when you almost crash your car—similar to an adrenaline rush. This could happen for two reasons. You could be sensitive to epinephrine (adrenaline) in the injection. Or the dentist administering the anesthetic could have inadvertently nicked or injected a blood vessel, bringing the epinephrine into the blood vessel too quickly. Fortunately, this rarely happens and is a temporary condition that typically dissipates rapidly.

WAKE UP TO A NEW SMILE: SEDATION DENTISTRY

In extreme cases, patients can be sedated for dental care. There is a huge contingency of dentophobics out there with broken-down smiles that are getting worse—all because of fear. Some of these people are well educated and affluent, so money is not the barrier. It's fear that keeps them out of the dental chair.

But once they're comfortable with the idea of being put to sleep and having their dentistry done while they're sleeping, they're ready to get in the chair and on the road to a healthy smile.

In my practice, we use two forms of sedation: a drug called triazolam, which is commonly known as Halcion (a common sleeping pill), and general anesthesia.

Triazolam. When triazolam (Halcion) is used in the dental office for sedation, you are asked not to eat or drink for eight hours before the appointment. One pill is given an hour before the appointment (obviously you need to be driven to and from the office) and another is given at the time you sit down in the chair.

Within fifteen minutes you feel the effect of the medication, which usually relaxes a nervous person enough that dentistry, including injections, can be done without causing any anxiety.

To ensure your safety, a monitoring device called a pulse oximeter measures heart rate, blood oxygen level, and blood pressure. Most people sleep through the procedure, but you can be woken intermittently when the dentist needs your cooperation to open or close your mouth to take a dental impression.

Triazolam is so safe and nontoxic that it would take a pill the size of a bowling ball for someone to overdose. In addition, there's a reversal agent that works immediately and can be administered in case of an emergency such as an adverse reaction or difficulty in breathing.

The other great benefit of this drug is that patients experience almost 100 percent amnesia, so when the procedure is finished, they go home feeling rested and have no memory of the entire visit.

I had a middle-aged dentophobic businessman who had been putting off having his mouth done for years. He heard about one of his friends who came in and had his whole smile made over under sedation, and that was all the impetus he needed. On the very first visit, I completed work on his upper and lower teeth. That evening, I called the patient to see how he was doing and he looked at the clock and said, "Oh, my God. Dr. Dorfman, I'm so sorry, I had an eight o'clock appointment with you this morning and it's nine o'clock. I missed it!"

I told him that it was nine o'clock p.m., not a.m., and that I had already done his mouth. He replied, "That's impossible." I told him to go look in the mirror. He came back, amazed, and said, "Doc, they're beautiful."

General anesthesia. For those who are even more apprehensive and want to be knocked out completely, many dentists use general anesthesia, administered by an anesthesiologist in the office. This is paramount to hospital dentistry.

With this kind of anesthesia, the patient is put to sleep with medication that is administered intravenously.

This treatment is reserved for patients who would never go to the dentist otherwise, because as with all anesthetics, there are always risks involved; in rare cases or if the anesthesia is not administered properly, the risks can be severe. That's why it's important to make sure that whoever is administering your anesthesia is properly certified and experienced. Under normal circumstances, this technique is not only safe and effective but also instrumental for normal maintenance and routine dental care.

Provided a patient can relax and take an injection of dental anesthetic, there is nothing that requires general anesthesia in dentistry. You name it—extractions, implants, root canals, and gum surgery have been performed for years on patients without general sedation. Today, the most common reason dental patients are given sedation is for extraction of their wisdom teeth. This has become de rigueur, but in reality it's unnecessary, and I advise against it unless the patient is dentophobic.

are you a teeth-whitening junkie?

5

blinded by the white

TEETH WHITENING

When it comes to teeth, bright and white is beautiful. According to the American Academy of Cosmetic Dentistry, the practice of teeth whitening (bleaching) has increased by more than 300 percent over the last several years. And bleaching is the number-one dental cosmetic procedure requested by patients under twenty *and* those twenty to fifty years old.

This chapter will help you sort through the avalanche of new teeth-whitening products now available from your dentist and over the counter. I'll save you a lot of time right now. None of those over-the-counter products are as safe and effective as the whitening treatment you'll receive through your cosmetic dentist. In fact, the tag line we use at Discus Dental—the world's largest manufacturer of tooth whitening products for dentists—is "Only a dentist can safely get your teeth their whitest."

Are you a teeth-whitening junkie? Remember the episode of *Friends* when Ross bleached his teeth so much they glowed in the dark? Don't worry, your teeth will never get *that* white. But it's always best to consult a dentist to confirm what shade will look best on your teeth.

Whitening teeth is an art and a science. Marketing wizards will tell you bleaching your teeth at home is as easy as coloring your hair. But absolutely do not try this at home without consulting a dentist first about what works best for you.

The bottom line: Not everyone is a good candidate for whitening, especially if you've had other cosmetic dentistry done. Let the professional decide. If you have dental restorations such as bonding, crowns, and veneers—unless you are willing to replace them with ones that are a lighter shade—then you are probably not the best candidate. But talk to your dentist and see what he or she can do.

I've seen it happen again and again—patients use store-bought products without regard to the bonding, crowns, or veneers on their teeth that do not change color. Even if their other teeth only change four to five shades, it no longer matches their bonding, crowns, or veneers, and it could cost thousands of dollars to make it match again. Remember, seeing a dentist *first* can prepare you for that sticker shock and give you the freedom to decide in advance which approach to take. And you'll avoid the cost of serious damage control. My personal mantra is "Inform before you perform."

the main causes of discolored teeth

Discolored teeth can result from various causes. These include

Genetics. Blame your parents for this one. Some people are just born with teeth that aren't particularly white.

Trauma. Teeth that have been broken, chipped, or hit in an accident can discolor. This is often a result of bleeding inside the tooth. Silver and composite fillings and root canal fillings can also discolor teeth.

External staining. Stains occur from smoking or drinking beverages such as coffee or tea, but these initially can just be polished off.

Aging. Because our teeth are porous, eventually superficial stains will penetrate and stain the actual tooth structure. The cause: a lifetime of smoking; drinking coffee, tea, red wine, and dark-colored soda and juices; and eating highly colored foods such as cherry pie, blueberries, soy sauce, and tomato sauce.

Medication. Some medication, such as tetracycline or fluoride, can cause internal gray stains or a gray, brown, or black banding on teeth. Children should *never* take any tetracycline derivative during the formative years of tooth development (usually up to age twelve to fourteen). As for adults, recent data shows that even fully formed adult teeth can gray with tetracycline, because of microcirculation of blood in the pulp of the teeth.

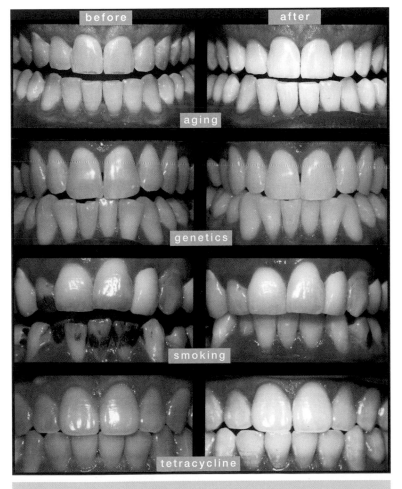

Bleaching results for stains caused by aging, genetics, smoking, and tetracycline.

choosing a color

It sounds like a silly question, but one of the first things I ask patients when they come in for a smile design consultation is "What color do you want your teeth?" Most respond "Uh, white?" or "Duh! White!" (Remember, I'm in Hollywood.) What you have to keep in mind is that there are a multitude of variations on white. It's somewhat like painting your living room white. You know from the paint store that there are a billion different shades of white: eggshell, satin, antique, white-white, and more.

Ten years ago, white was either shade A1 or B1 from the Vita Shade Guide, which is the most common standard shade guide for dentists. However, with the popularity of bleaching, today those shades would be considered too dark by most. In fact, I don't know of a single young celebrity in Hollywood who would accept A1 or B1 as a light enough shade for their teeth.

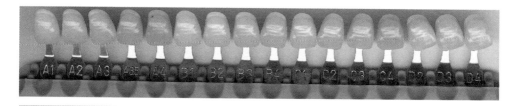

Standard Vita Shade Guide, which is used by dentists to measure shades of teeth.

The new standard for whiteness is typically a natural bleach shade. This is the color of a natural tooth that has been bleached, but it is not as white as Ross's teeth looked on *Friends*. On *Extreme Makeover*, I usually use an A1 shade of porcelain blended with a bleached shade to create a color slightly lighter than natural light teeth. This method renders the teeth into a bleached but still natural shade.

However, if a patient comes in and wants the most natural smile possible—and I mean the kind of natural that is completely undetectable even to a dentist—then I'd use an A1 shade or a shade slightly lighter than A1, because that's the lightest that natural teeth can be without bleaching.

Some patients will come in and say, "Doc, I want my teeth really white, like Regis Philbin white." You have to understand, a seventeen-year-old will naturally have really white teeth, but it's impossible for a seventy-year-old man or woman to have teeth that bright—at least not naturally. Although tooth whitening can often reverse the process of staining and create a shade comparable to that of someone in his or her teens, this color does not look natural on an older person. But even though it's not always age-appropriate or natural, it's not uncommon for patients to want that snow-white shade anyway. And many dentists do it. They feel that what the patient wants, the patient should get, even though the dentists may know better.

With that being said, there is a natural limit to how white your teeth can get. When you see people whose teeth are absurdly white, 99.9 percent of the time it is because they've had unnaturally white bonding, veneers, or crowns made. It is virtually impossible to bleach natural teeth to the point where they look fake—if teeth look fake, chances are they are fake.

Healthy yellow teeth (shade A2–A3.5 from the Vita Shade Guide) respond best to tooth whitening products. Yellow is the best jumping-off point; darker gray, brown, and black hues are actually tougher to whiten. If you have darker teeth, you may need to use take-home trays from your dentist for several weeks to months for optimal results (see page 118).

There are some general guidelines for choosing a natural-looking shade of white, based on complexion and hair color. If you have a fair complexion with light-colored eyes and hair, then you should choose a brighter shade of white. Stay away from a white with any yellow in it because the yellow will look even more yellow without the contrast of dark skin.

In turn, the darker your skin, the brighter your smile will appear. It all has to do with contrast. So if you have a dark complexion, don't pick a color that is super-white, because it will look even whiter on you. Similarly, for people with dark hair, I go with a more muted natural hue of white.

Gray-haired people are treated as if they were blonde, so choose a whiter shade if your hair is gray.

If your hair is a reddish hue, stay away from yellow shades. For you, it's white all the way.

Whatever your coloring, you want a shade that is not unnaturally white and is age-appropriate. Consider eye color an accent and don't let it influence your tooth shade much. People sometimes come in and ask if their teeth should match the whiteness of their eyes. Even some dentists think there's a correlation between the colors. What does one have to do with the other? I don't see the connection at all. If both your eyes and teeth are yellow, you have two problems. We can fix *one* of them.

The best way to determine the right shade for you is to have your dentist fabricate a set of temporaries in the shade you selected and take 'em out for a test drive. Because as difficult as it is for a dentist to look at a shade tab and determine if it works for you, it's even more difficult for you as a patient.

whitening methods

You have three basic whitening methods to choose from: dentist-supervised take-home trays with whitening gel, in-office whitening treatment, and over-the-counter whitening products.

TAKE-HOME TRAYS

After a thorough cleaning and oral examination, your dental professional will help you determine if you are a good candidate for whitening. Whitening is ideal for patients who have healthy, natural teeth. If you have any pre-existing cosmetic restorations (bonding, porcelain, crowns, or veneers), because these won't bleach, you may need to replace them once you have completed whitening treatment in order to match your new white smile. Whitening is not recommended for anyone who is pregnant or nursing—we actually don't know that there are any adverse effects, but no studies have been done to verify this.

Once you and your dental professional decide which tooth whitening option is best for you, the process is easy. For take-home trays, a whitening gel is placed in an inconspicuous, clear tray that comfortably fits over your teeth. As the hydrogen peroxide in the gel breaks down, oxygen enters the enamel and dentin to lighten discolorations. The structure is not changed; only the color is made lighter. Results are usually noticed after the very first application, and maximum results generally occur after three to fourteen days of treatment.

On your first visit. Impressions of your teeth are taken so that a custom-fitted whitening tray can be made. The dental office will let you know when you can pick up your trays and whitening gel. In some cases, the dental office may be able to have your trays ready on the same visit.

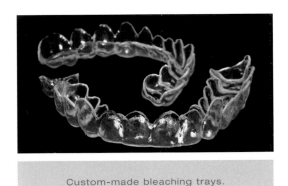

Custom-made bleaching trays.

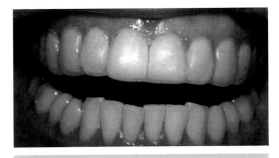

Bleaching tray filled with gel and positioned on the upper teeth.

On the next visit. Once you have been comfortably fitted with your whitening trays, your dental professional uses a shade guide to indicate the current color of your teeth. This will let you see how many shades you have lightened at the completion of the whitening process. At this appointment, you may be asked to choose between whitening during the day or overnight while you sleep. While at home, be sure to follow the take-home whitening instructions and always follow the advice of your dental professional. And if you notice white spots, don't panic—they are due to dehydration and will go away in a week or two (if they were not present before bleaching). Some patients also experience some sensitivity, but that disappears within a couple of days (see page 122).

Pros of take-home trays:	Cons of take-home trays:
> Produce white teeth	> Occasional temporary sensitivity
> Can be used at your convenience	> Occasional temporary white spots
> When administered by a dentist, they are safe, fast, and effective	> Take three to fourteen days for full effect
	> Bonding, veneers, or crowns may have to be replaced to match your new color
	> Patient compliance is critical for success

ZOOM! YOUR WAY TO WHITE TEETH

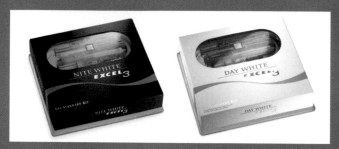

Nite White and Day White dentist-dispensed whitening kits.

Of course, I'm partial to my own teeth-whitening products. Discus Dental revolutionized dentistry by adding sex appeal to the industry. I said, "Why not market teeth-whitening products like cosmetics?" Make-up can only mask so much, but beautiful teeth are essential to making your face light up.

We at Discus Dental believe that tooth whitening should be done or supervised by a dentist. Our first two whitening products were dentist-dispensed take-home tray systems. Nite White is a pleasant-tasting gel that's placed in a custom-fitted tray and worn overnight while you sleep. Day White is a tray system that uses a fast-acting gel that is placed in a tray for thirty minutes twice a day. Both are used for three to fourteen days.

But if you need that killer smile faster, take a seat in your dentist's chair and let the ZOOM! light work its magic. The ZOOM! Chairside Whitening System is an advanced tooth-whitening procedure that is safe, effective, and convenient. And in less than one hour your teeth will become dramatically whiter.

A study has shown that use of the ZOOM! lamp increases the effectiveness of the ZOOM! gel by 26 percent or more over just gel use in trays. ZOOM! will produce an average improvement of eight shades in under an hour.

With proper care your smile will sparkle for years.

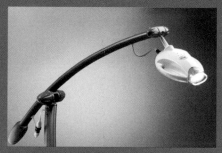

ZOOM! lamp.

IN-OFFICE WHITENING

Take-home trays are fine, but if you just can't wait and you're really pressed for time—and you have to have your new, white smile yesterday—your dentist can use an in-office whitening treatment to make your teeth up to ten shades lighter in just under an hour.

It may be called "chairside bleaching," and usually a special light is used to activate a bleaching agent that is carefully applied to your teeth. Once lasers were used, but now most procedures are light activated.

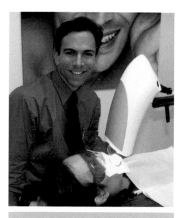

A patient undergoes ZOOM! treatment in my office.

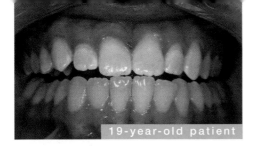
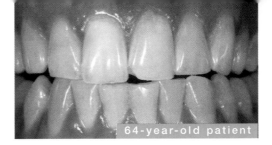

19-year-old patient

64-year-old patient

To demonstrate the dramatic effect of the in-office whitening process, these patients had ZOOM! whitening on the upper arch only. The left photo was taken three months after treatment; the right photo was taken six months after treatment.

The procedure begins with covering your lips, mouth, and gums to protect them, leaving only your teeth exposed. In our office the lips and mouth are covered with napkins and gauze, while the gums are covered with a protective "paint-on" resin that is cured with the same light we use in bonding. A bleaching agent is applied, and then the light is used. The light and gel work together to gently penetrate your teeth, breaking up stains and discoloration.

Here's how it works. The light activates the gel's active ingredient, either hydrogen peroxide, carbamide peroxide, or a combination of the two. As the peroxide is broken down, oxygen enters the enamel and dentin, bleaching colored substances while the structure of the tooth is unchanged. In addition to activating the hydrogen peroxide, the light helps it penetrate the surface of the tooth. While you sit back and relax, the gel is applied. In our ZOOM! procedure, this is done for three fifteen-minute cycles.

As with take-home trays, some patients experience sensitivity or white spots due to dehydration; fortunately, these side effects are only temporary. Sensitivity always disappears within a day or two; any white spot (that was not present before bleaching) will disappear in a week or two after bleaching.

Pros of in-office whitening treatment:	Cons of in-office whitening treatment:
> Produces white teeth	> Occasional temporary sensitivity
> Immediate results, usually in forty-five minutes to an hour	> Occasional temporary white spots
> Easy	> Somewhat more expensive than trays
> Patient compliance is not a factor, since the dentist does the treatment	> May need to have bonding, veneers, or crowns replaced to match your new color

OVER-THE-COUNTER WHITENING PRODUCTS

Over-the-counter (OTC) whitening products include toothpaste, strips, gels, paint-on products and liquids, and some that claim to be light activated. Granted, some of these products will work to a certain extent, but I maintain that for the best results you should see your dentist. These OTC products themselves simply aren't as effective as the products your dentist carries; furthermore, they will not offer the guidance you can get from your dentist, and will not be customized for your needs.

DEALING WITH SENSITIVITY

Sensitivity from whitening can range from mild to severe. In some cases, your dentist may prescribe Motrin or a strong pain relief medication to combat the pain. It's unusual for the pain to last more than a few hours. Even better news: The pain rarely lasts through the night and always does go away. Many dentists and scientists have developed theories as to why this sensation occurs, but all we know for sure is that the nerve becomes temporarily inflamed, and that it is never permanent.

Most of the new whitening gels use sensitivity agents such as fluoride (to reduce hydrostatic pressure) and potassium nitrate (the active ingredient in most desensitizing toothpastes) to block nerve conduction. Discus products also use amorphous calcium phosphate (ACP) to help remineralize teeth and combat sensitivity. Personally, I can use only our take-home products Nite White and Day White with ACP, as my teeth are sensitive to other whitening gels.

Toothpastes. The best you can expect from a "whitening toothpaste" is that it will remove some light superficial stains on your teeth. No toothpaste can change the color of the tooth structure, however.

Gels. Because whitening gels are not regulated, you have no assurance that they are effective or safe. While most use the same ingredients as the professional systems, they are not as strong and usually do not work as well. One of the biggest problems with OTC whiteners is that some are made too acidic in order to stabilize them, which can cause permanent damage to the surface of your teeth. Professional products have a neutral pH so they are safe.

Strips. Strips can work unevenly and they brighten only the front six teeth. Most people show at least twelve upper teeth when they smile, however, so unless you also use bleaching trays, the back teeth will remain dark. And unlike the specialized bleaching trays provided at your dentist's office, over-the-counter strips and trays aren't custom-made for your smile. This means that if you have rotated teeth, or larger or smaller than average teeth, the store-bought strips or trays will not fit properly and you can end up with a botched, uneven whitening job.

Paint-on products and liquids. The key to efficacy is contact time. The active ingredient must have prolonged exposure to work, unless a light or laser is used to accelerate the process. These products are just not very effective.

OTC light-activated products. These products make claims, but I have not been impressed with their data. Lots of sizzle, no steak.

Pros of OTC whitening products:	Cons of OTC whitening products:
> May not be as expensive as products or services from your dentist > Convenient to purchase; can be an impulse buy	> Not as effective as professional products > No guarantees > Not custom made or custom selected for your teeth > Safety is not assured > No professional guidance: not every patient is a good candidate for whitening > May need to have bonding, veneers, or crowns replaced to match your new color

maintaining your white smile

To maintain that brilliantly bright new smile, you have to brush, floss, and continue to see your dentist for routine checkups and cleanings.

How long does whitening last? Every case is different. It depends on the physical make-up of your teeth and your lifestyle. But to keep that smile bright, you should do touchups every six months or so with the take-home trays your dentist made. Just a night

REPLACING OLD FILLINGS THAT DISCOLOR TEETH

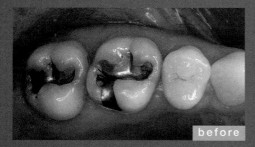
before

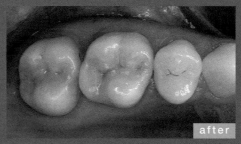
after

Old silver fillings in this patient's molars caused dark stains. The silver fillings were removed and replaced with bonded composite fillings, giving the teeth a more natural appearance.

Silver fillings (amalgams) can discolor teeth because they tend to allow moisture to leak in, which turns the tooth even darker. Also, amalgam expands as it sets, and unfortunately, this expansion never stops! Over time, because of this continual expansion especially large fillings may cause teeth to crack; the larger the filling, the more it will expand and the greater the chance the tooth will crack. They may eventually even cause tooth death, which means you will need root canals, crowns, or—in a worst-case scenario—implants to replace your teeth. By replacing the old silver fillings with tooth-colored composite resin or porcelain, the natural color of the tooth can be restored and the tooth structure will be reinforced. Porcelain fillings make the tooth stronger, not weaker.

Even though the new tooth-colored restorations cost more than traditional metal fillings, they are stronger and more aesthetic, and do not contain the dreaded mercury found in silver amalgam. I have refused to use silver amalgams for over twenty years because of the mercury, and you should insist that your dentist do only amalgam-free dentistry!

or two every now and then will revive that sparkle. If you're a smoker or heavy coffee or red wine drinker, you may need to do it more often than that.

Again, everyone's teeth are different, and some are more porous and susceptible to staining than others, so the length of time that whitening lasts varies on a case-by-case basis. I've had some patients who still look good five years after their whitening without any touchups at all, and others who need to touch up for a night or two every few months.

only floss
the teeth
you want
to keep

6

let's keep
it clean, folks

HYGIENE AND PREVENTION

So now that you have a beautiful smile, how do you maintain it? Think about the day you picked up your new car. Remember how shiny and perfect it looked? Remember how it smelled? More importantly, do you recall how good you felt driving it home?

What does that car look and smell like now? Probably nothing like when it was new!

Your new smile is like a new car. It will require constant upkeep to stay fresh and new looking.

In this chapter I outline my dental care tips. My MO is a very simple, back-to-basics approach: Brush and floss regularly and see your dentist for regular checkups. Easy, right? But many people neglect these three simple things, inviting a host of dental problems they could have avoided. And if you are concerned about your breath, I would follow the brush and floss, scrape, and rinse regime.

Plaque is the enemy! That sticky film of bacteria causes tooth decay and gum disease. Although experts say you should brush and floss twice a day, I say stay on the offensive and brush and floss after every meal to keep plaque at bay.

Many patients think that because nothing hurts they don't have to go to the dentist.

That's a painful way to live—and can lead to lasting damage. By the time something hurts, it is typically too late. Visit your dental hygienist or dentist at least every six months.

brushing

As you'll see in my brushing tips, you should always brush gently over the outer and the inner surfaces and over the chewing surfaces of the teeth. But go easy! Just because you had a hard day, don't take your aggressions out on your teeth. If you brush too hard, you can actually wear your enamel and dentin away, and cause permanent damage to your gums. Once gums recede, they never come back.

Always use a soft brush. This goes for everyone, from age nine to ninety! Why do they even sell hard brushes? They destroy teeth—you might as well be brushing with sandpaper!

Don't get too attached to that toothbrush either. It takes only a few months for your brush to wear out and become ineffective. You should replace it every two to three months.

It's important to brush your gums as well as your teeth to prevent bad breath and periodontal disease. Be gentle because your gums are very sensitive. Brush the area where the tooth meets the gums. Don't waste time brushing your tongue. (To most effectively remove the bacteria that cause bad breath, it's best to scrape your tongue with a tongue scraper—more on this later.)

Experts estimate the toothbrush dates back to around AD 1000 in China. Back then it was called a "chew stick" and it was believed to have been made from hog's bristles. It wasn't until the 1930s that synthetic materials were used in toothbrushes. Up until thirty years ago, it was all about hard bristles because it was widely believed that the harder you brushed, the cleaner your teeth would be.

If you use a manual toothbrush, you should brush for between three to five minutes. With a power brush, two minutes does the job. However, most manual users spend only twenty-four to sixty seconds on their entire oral hygiene routine. And they brush incorrectly as well! Not you, of course, dear reader.

HOW TO CLEAN YOUR MOUTH PROPERLY

> Place the toothbrush at a forty-five-degree angle against your gums.

> Rotate the brush gently in small, circular motions.

> Brush the outer surfaces of each tooth on both the upper and lower arches.

> Repeat on the inside surfaces and chewing surfaces of all teeth.

> Scrape the tongue with a tongue scraper to remove bad-breath-causing bacteria. Move it from the back of the tongue toward the front, sweeping the bacteria out of the mouth.

> Rinse with water or alcohol-free mouthwash.

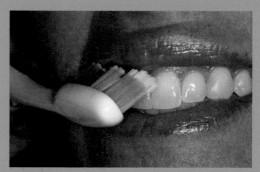

Hold a soft toothbrush at a forty-five-degree angle to the gums and gently rotate it into the gumline.

POWER TOOTHBRUSHES

I use one. Enough said! It's a choice every brusher has to make: to let the brush do the brushing or to give your wrist a workout.

Studies show that power brushes appear to be superior to manual brushes. More plaque can be removed in less time, and built-in timers (usually two minutes) are great because most people don't brush long enough. Another advantage is that with a power brush you have to concern yourself only with where the brush goes, not how to brush—especially good for those who need to improve their brushing technique.

My favorite brush is Sonicare by Philips, equipped with a built-in two-minute timer. Ultimately, the Sonicare toothbrush can do in two minutes what it would take you to do in four to six minutes with a manual toothbrush. Whatever brand you choose, the toothbrush should be comfortable and not too aggressive, because it could cause damage to your teeth and gums.

But no matter how good a brusher you are, you're not a professional dental hygienist, so regular visits to the dentist (at least every six months) will make sure that plaque and calculus (tartar) buildup are under control. Long-term neglect can lead to subgingival (under the gums) accumulation of plaque and calculus, which harbor bacteria that destroy the bone supporting your teeth. The eventual result could be bad breath, periodontal disease, and ultimately tooth loss.

CHOOSING A TOOTHPASTE

The toothpaste aisle seems to be growing bigger and bigger. There are so many choices: fluoride, whitening, fluoride with whitening, and more. Whether you like baking soda or mint sparkles in your toothpaste is up to you. Keep in mind that the most important ingredient is still fluoride!

As mentioned earlier, whitening toothpastes are more and more popular, but they don't actually whiten teeth once and for all. I want to dispel one big white lie (pun intended): *Toothpaste doesn't whiten teeth.* Brushing with toothpaste may remove or brush away superficial or surface stains, such as coffee, tea, or tar and nicotine on a smoker's teeth, thus making the teeth appear lighter. However, the actual tooth structure has not become lighter. Real bleaching takes more than the few minutes brushing can provide. To my knowledge, no clinical evidence supports the claims so-called whitening toothpastes make to actually lighten tooth structure. If these toothpastes were drugs, the manufacturers would have to substantiate their claims to the FDA, but because they're not categorized as drugs, manufacturers can make vague claims that can be misleading.

Buyer beware! Some of these so-called whitening toothpastes tend to be too abrasive and over years of use can wear away the enamel on your teeth. So check with your dentist before using this type of toothpaste. Remember, avoiding abrasive toothpaste is critical in preventing tooth destruction. Using abrasive toothpaste actually "sands" or wears away your enamel. This causes irreversible tooth damage, which will require bonding or porcelain crowns or veneers to repair. Unfortunately, there's no way of knowing how abrasive a toothpaste is until you try it. If it feels too grainy or sandy while brushing, chances are it's too abrasive.

By the way, the same thing goes for teeth-whitening chewing gum, which also does not whiten teeth. However, there is evidence that chewing sugarless gum can help fight plaque buildup by generating saliva flow, which helps wash plaque away.

THE POWER OF FLUORIDE

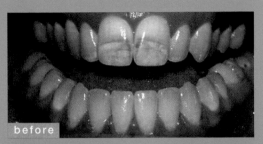
before

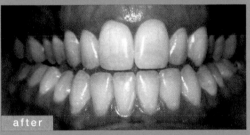
after

These teeth had brown and white stains from too much fluoride. Fortunately for this patient, a two-week course of take-home whitening with Nite White removed the stains. Some patients are not so lucky.

Fluoride is key to fighting plaque. Once it's incorporated into the tooth structure, it strengthens the tooth, making it less permeable and more resistant to cavities. It's in most city water systems and in most toothpastes. But if you're a fan of bottled water, keep in mind that most do not contain fluoride—check the labels. If you drink unfluoridated bottled water, if your city does not provide fluoridated water, or if you have well water, ask your dentist or pediatrician if you should take fluoride supplements.

Whether or not children should take fluoride substitutes is a tricky question. Fluoride you ingest during the years your teeth are forming will become permanently incorporated into the tooth structure. This is even more effective in strengthening teeth and making them less prone to cavities than the topical fluoride in toothpaste. However, if a child consumes too much fluoride, it can permanently scar the adult teeth with white or brown spots. If you are lucky, brown spots can be bleached or sanded off by a dentist.

Fluoride's one of those cases where too little or too much won't do the job—it has to be just right.

flossing

Patients always ask me, "Doc, do I really need to floss my teeth?" And I always tell them, "Only floss the teeth you want to keep!"

Flossing is an acquired skill. It takes practice. While many consider it to be a pain in the you-know-what, flossing is a must. It removes plaque between the teeth that toothbrushes simply cannot reach and stimulates the gums. Stimulating the gums keeps them healthy and tight; this helps prevent plaque from setting up shop in your mouth and manufacturing bacteria. Enough said. At a minimum, floss every night before you go to bed. (As I mentioned earlier, I floss after every meal.)

If you don't floss, you could end up like one of my close friends and the king of all cavities, Sean Astin. I tease because I love the guy! He is a great guy and one fantastic actor. You might have seen him as an aspiring Notre Dame football player in *Rudy,* as a hobbit in *The Lord of the Rings,* or playing a counter-terrorist government agent on the television show *24.* Sean is Hollywood royalty, the son of actors Patty Duke (from whom I bought my first house) and John Astin.

Sean and I appeared on *The View* together and he confessed that he never flosses. So in jest I said, "Sean, that's how I pay my mortgage—because people like you never floss!" The women on *The View* got a kick out of that one. But there is some truth to it.

If people flossed more, many of them wouldn't need to spend so much of their hard-earned money on dental treatment. Flossing really does make a difference. But you have to be diligent about it. It's simply something you have to do at least before you go to bed at night.

If you're a novice flosser or you floss only now and then, you may notice that your gums bleed a little while flossing. That's just your body's way of telling you that you aren't flossing enough, and it should stop pretty quickly once you're flossing daily. But see your dentist if your gums continue to bleed even when you're brushing and flossing on a regular basis.

HOW TO FLOSS PROPERLY

> Pull out about fifteen to twenty inches of floss, winding most of it around the middle fingers of both hands.

> Hold the floss lightly between the thumbs and forefingers.

> Use a gentle back and forth motion to guide the floss between the teeth. Once you've gotten the floss past where the teeth touch each other, switch to a gentle up and down motion.

> When you reach the gums, stop! Never "saw" into the gum tissue or you will destroy it. Instead, use an up and down motion.

> Advance the floss so you continually use a fresh section of the floss.

> Repeat this procedure on each tooth—even in the back!

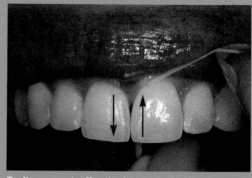

To floss most effectively, wrap the floss around each tooth and move up and down, *not* back and forth

why you want to brush and floss

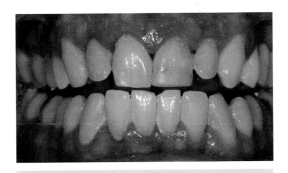

Redness of the gums around the teeth is a sign of gingivitis.

Periodontal disease (periodontitis) occurs when the gum tissues and bones that hold the teeth in place deteriorate. Worst-case scenario, left untreated it can result in tooth loss.

What causes periodontal disease? Usually the cause is plaque and the toxins produced by plaque—which you can control with careful daily brushing and flossing and regular dental visits. Plaque hardens into calculus (tartar), which harbors damaging bacteria in the gums and around your teeth. Other times it is the result of injury, medication, or just bleeding gums.

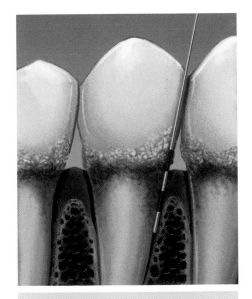

Plaque and calculus buildup on teeth can cause bone loss. Here a probe with markers is being used to measure bone loss.

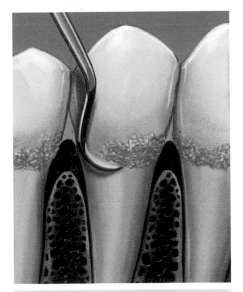

The dental hygienist uses an instrument called a scaler to remove the debris that builds up on your teeth.

Symptoms of periodontal disease include bleeding gums (yes, they can be both a cause and a symptom!), pus between the teeth and gums, loose teeth, and persistent bad breath. If left untreated it will result in infection and tooth loss.

Gingivitis is a mild form of gum disease, where your gums become swollen and bleed a bit but there are no other problems or discomfort. Gingivitis, left untreated, can advance to periodontitis, when bone loss begins to occur. But unlike periodontitis, gingivitis can be reversible when you and your dentist team up and fight it together.

Because gingivitis is often just the result of poor oral hygiene, it can be avoided if you take care of yourself, your teeth, and your gums.

scraping the tongue

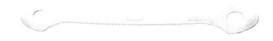

BreathRx tongue scraper by Discus Dental.

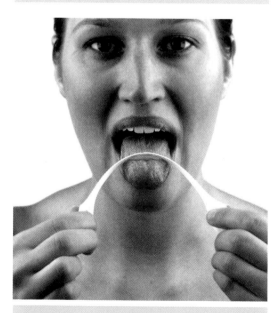

When scraping the tongue, move the scraper from the back of the tongue toward the front of the mouth and then out.

Here's the bad news: Clinical research shows that 90 percent of bad breath originates on the surface of the tongue. Unfortunately, using your toothbrush to brush your tongue only moves around the bacteria that cause bad breath (also called biofilm) and can even carry the bacteria to other sites in the mouth.

Now here's the good news: A tongue scraper can come to the rescue! Sold in the toothbrush section of most drugstores, a tongue scraper can literally sweep those bacteria out of your mouth.

Daily tongue scraping is the best five to ten seconds you can spend on your breath. Period. I consider the BreathRx tongue scraper from Discus Dental ideal for this. To get the most out of tongue scraping, use the BreathRx tongue spray first. It will kill the bacteria and loosen it from all those crevices on the tongue, making the scraping even more effective and long lasting. (For more on BreathRx products, see www.discus-dental.com or www.BreathRx.com.)

When scraping your tongue, it's important to move the scraper from the back of the tongue, where most of the foul-smelling bad-breath bacteria live, toward the front of the mouth and then out. Rinse with water or an alcohol-free mouthwash such as BreathRx afterwards.

Your loved ones and colleagues will thank you, and you may enjoy your food more, because tongue scraping is believed to heighten the sensitivity of taste buds. This oral hygiene habit is probably the most effective for maintaining fresh breath and optimal oral health! (For more information on fighting bad breath, see Chapter 7.)

cavities

You knew it was coming, didn't you?

Cavities are little craters that form in your teeth because of decay. A cavity will eat right through the hard enamel surface (the white, visible part of your teeth) into the dentin and eventually the pulp. That's when it can cause an abscess, and the infection and swelling can be severe. At this point,

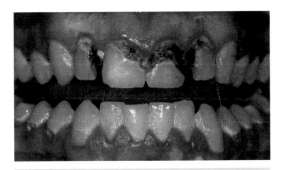

This patient had gross decay due to poor oral hygiene and too much soda consumption.

there is usually a lot of pain and the only hope to save your tooth is to have a root canal.

The infection can spread into the tooth's blood vessels and create an abscess in the tooth's roots. If you haven't seen a dentist by the time that happens, then you're in for a shock, because the pain can be unbearable.

CAUSES OF CAVITIES

You can blame bacteria for cavities. When bacteria build up on teeth that are not brushed or flossed regularly, they produce an acid that literally eats away at the tooth.

Sometimes cavities are tough to control. Once the decay starts, it rarely stops; if left untreated, it burrows right into the nerve until—you guessed it. You need a root canal.

Here are some clues that you might have a cavity:

> Pain, pain, pain
> Heightened sensitivity to hot and cold drinks
> Bad breath (worse than just morning breath)
> Black or brown pits

TREATMENT OF CAVITIES

Getting yourself to a dentist is the first step if you think you're getting a cavity. Your dentist will remove all traces of decay in your tooth with a drill, laser, or abrasion unit. Don't worry, your dentist will offer you an anesthetic, so you won't feel a thing. Then your tooth will be filled with either a metal or a composite tooth-colored filling that will hopefully save your tooth. I recommend tooth-colored restorations not only because they look better, but because they are usually better for your teeth—metal fillings expand and can eventually crack your teeth, while the composite fillings do not expand and actually hold your tooth together.

Just remember, cavities are *totally* avoidable and you can get them at any age. So take care for life!

HOW TO AVOID CAVITIES

> Brush and floss regularly.
> Use a fluoride toothpaste.
> Avoid snacking between meals without brushing.
> Visit your dentist for regular checkups.

helping your kids develop good dental routines

Even babies can start early toward good dental health—even before birth. If you're pregnant, get lots of calcium because your baby's teeth develop between the third and sixth months. And you should brush your child's teeth and gums with baby toothpaste and a baby toothbrush or finger cot when you see that first baby tooth. Don't use fluoride toothpaste on babies' teeth—and a child should not use fluoride toothpaste until he or she learns how to spit. Otherwise they will ingest too much fluoride.

I don't think it's important for toddlers to learn how to brush their teeth. You should do it for them. Even though these are only baby teeth and your child will eventually lose them, you don't want them to be lost prematurely. This could negatively affect the proper spacing and skeletal position of their permanent teeth. Infections from decay in baby teeth could also permanently damage adult teeth.

So brush your young child's teeth just as you would your own: up, down, gentle circles at the gum line. Make sure you cover every surface of every tooth. But go easy. A child's mouth can be much more sensitive than an adult's, so you don't want to brush too hard. Fluoride is critical for your child's teeth, so select a children's toothpaste that contains fluoride and tastes good, so they will allow you to brush longer.

In my opinion, flossing is not necessary until permanent teeth come in because there is usually enough space between children's teeth to allow a toothbrush to reach in and clean and stimulate the gums. Most children have a complete set of teeth by approximately twelve or thirteen years old.

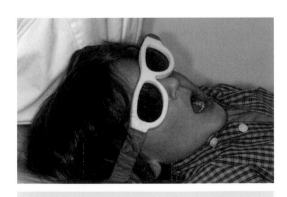

Taking children to the dentist at an early age helps develop a healthy oral hygiene regimen.

Taking your children to the dentist early is like putting them in car seats right away. So start regular dental checkups as soon as their teeth grow in, around age one. If they learn to accept it at an early enough age, they'll be set for life.

protecting your teeth

Besides careful brushing and flossing, there are other things you can do to help protect your teeth.

SEALANTS

Sealants are recommended for children and for adults who are prone to cavities. Decay is most prevalent in the back teeth (premolars and molars) because that's where deep grooves form on the biting surfaces. Plaque collects in these grooves and causes cavities. To keep healthy teeth cavity free, sealants can be applied to the chewing

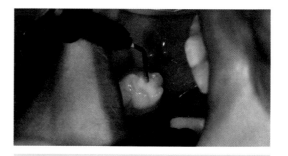

Sealant is being applied to this child's tooth.

surfaces. This prevents bacteria from sticking around long enough to cause damage, thus keeping teeth cavity free on the surface.

Sealing teeth is quick and easy. A dentist simply brushes the quick-drying light-cured liquid sealant onto the teeth, shines a light on it and presto—it hardens on top of

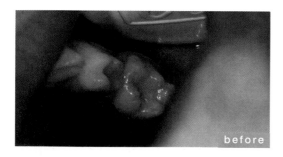
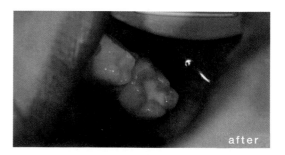

before

after

Sealant was applied to these teeth to prevent plaque from collecting in the deep grooves.

the teeth. And it's pain free. Plus, for the several years it lasts, it prevents the painful experience of cavities.

During routine checkups, ask the dentist to check to make sure sealants have not or will not become dislodged. As long as they stay intact, sealants will prevent cavities from forming on the chewing surface.

But remember, sealants do not prevent decay between the teeth; only fluoride and flossing can do this.

This proactive approach can protect vulnerable teeth from "plaque attack." It's not unlike investing in vinyl siding for your house. But it's relatively inexpensive and it protects the tooth underneath for many years to come.

SNORING

The American Dental Association estimates between 10 and 30 percent of adults snore. You probably know who you are and whoever shares a bed with you knows who you are for sure! They probably wished they didn't. Believe it or not, your dentist can help with a variety of oral appliances, such as plastic snore guards that position the jaw and improve breathing. These devices work by moving the lower jaw forward—much like they teach in CPR training—to better open up the airway.

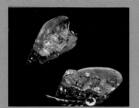 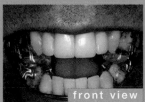 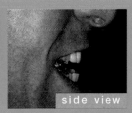

front view

side view

I volunteered to model this snore guard. In the side view, notice how my lower jaw is pushed forward and open. This opens up the airway, much like the position used in CPR does.

MOUTH GUARDS

When I was a kid we didn't wear helmets when we rode our bikes around the neighborhood. It's amazing I survived childhood at all! But now even adults wear helmets for biking, skiing, and a multitude of sports. The International Academy for Sports Dentistry recommends wearing a mouth guard during sports to protect your smile. And you don't have to be a linebacker to lose a few teeth. Children playing contact sports and weekend warriors fall flat on their faces all the time.

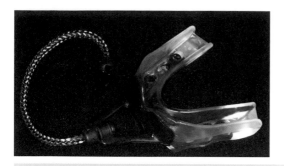
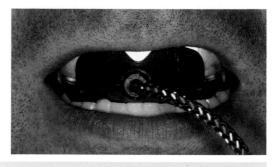

Depending on the sport, athletic mouth guards cover both upper and lower teeth (left) or only upper teeth (right). Some have helmet straps, as shown.

To protect yourself, ask your dentist to custom-fit a mouth guard made for your teeth, whether your sport is bicycling, inline skating, racquetball, baseball, hockey, football, basketball, or boxing—and do the same for your children. Mouth guards found in sporting good stores are usually fine to use for sports, but show them to your dentist before using.

Let the mouth guard absorb the blows, not your teeth!

AVOIDING TEETH GRINDING

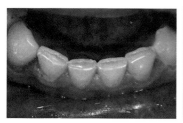
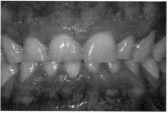
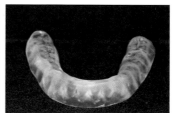
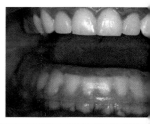

This patient had excessive wear on the lower front teeth and the upper front teeth due to teeth grinding.

A custom-made night guard worn on either the upper or lower arch can help prevent teeth grinders from damaging their teeth.

The American Dental Association calls it bruxism. Teeth grinding is a problem many people don't realize they have because they may do it only while they're asleep. But they notice the symptoms when they wake up in the morning: Headaches, toothaches, and sore facial muscles are dead giveaways that you're a grinder. And excessive wear on your teeth is confirmation.

A variety of reasons, such as stress, behavior, genetics, or even an abnormal bite, could cause you to grind your teeth. If you're not sure you grind, the person you sleep with may hear or see you doing it. Or ask a dentist, who can identify the problem by looking for wear marks on your teeth. I've had many patients swear they don't grind or have "stopped" grinding their teeth, and they are almost *always* wrong.

Chances are, if you have wear patterns, you grind—if so, you probably will never stop. To protect your teeth from grinding, your dentist can outfit you with a custom-

THE CONNECTION BETWEEN HEADACHES AND SMILES

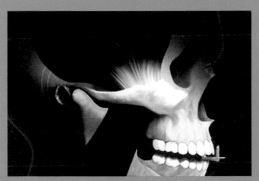
A schematic diagram shows how the Best-Bite appliance positions the lower jaw for optimal muscle relaxation.

The newest studies have shown that some head, neck, and facial pain is caused or triggered by the jaw muscles. It's easy to see how this could be: Just place your hands on the side of your face and clench your teeth together—you can feel the big jaw muscles all the way from your cheeks to your temples.

Most leading dentists agree that an uneven bite can frequently trigger teeth clenching and grinding. This in turn can cause worn-down teeth, which are often treated with porcelain veneers and crowns. But for many years, the underlying problem, the uneven bite, has been overlooked, especially in the case of people with head, neck, and facial pain.

The problem is that when a person's bite is not even, it's somewhat like trying to walk with one shoe on and one shoe off. It can be done, but other muscles have to overwork to compensate. And that extra muscle activity can cause the muscles to fatigue and start to hurt. These overworked muscles can cause primary pain or can trigger secondary pain such as tension and migraine headaches.

Some patients seek chiropractic care or physical therapy to work on the muscles. But unless the bite is corrected and the jaw balanced, the muscles will not relax.

Until recently, it has been difficult to diagnose and treat head, neck, and facial pain caused by an uneven bite. However, a new device, the Best-Bite Discluder, takes much of the mystery and technical difficulty out of the process. This device works quickly, easily, and inexpensively to center the jaw joints and put them in balance, and let the muscles relax at the same time.

If your pain is caused by your bite, the pain stops in less than two minutes. You get a diagnosis and relief at the same time! This device has zero side effects, does not cause drowsiness or stomach upset like drugs, and can be used at any time at the onset of any head, neck, and facial pain. (You can find more info at www.best-bite.com.)

You can use it as a rescue device for just a few minutes at a time, as needed, to relieve the muscles to stop the pain. People use it one or two times a day or just a couple of times a week to stop the muscle spasm and break the cycle of pain. (With a long-lasting silicone liner, you can use it hundreds of times.) Realizing that their problem has been an uneven bite, many people who experience relief with this device choose to get their bite fixed by their dentist for permanent pain relief.

made night guard. Grinding can destroy an entire set of teeth and cost tens of thousands of dollars to repair. So please wear a night guard if your dentist prescribes one. It's so much easier to replace your night guard every few years than all your teeth! (Note that over-the-counter mouth guards sold for sports protection are not suitable for teeth grinders; only a custom-fit guard from your dentist will keep your jaw in place and thus prevent grinding and wear-down.)

When Marilyn Monroe was once asked what she wore to bed, she said, "Only Chanel No. 5." For grinders, I say, "All you *need* to wear to bed is your night guard."

how diet affects dental health

Research suggests that your diet affects your dental health. While periodontal disease isn't necessarily caused by a poor diet, research suggests it progresses faster with a nutrient-poor diet.

Just like most things in life, it's all about common sense. Sugar and starch help cause cavities, while vegetables are good for your entire body, not just your teeth.

Vitamins B, C, D, and E all help keep gums healthy and fight gingivitis, gum inflammation that can progress to gum disease. You can find these vitamins in fresh fruits and vegetables. If you're not getting enough in your daily diet, take supplements.

Calcium is also very important to maintain healthy teeth and bones, especially your jawbone, which holds that beautiful new smile in place! Milk isn't the only place to get calcium. Tofu, soy, nuts, broccoli, kale, and spinach are also rich in calcium.

Foods, gum, and mints that contain xylitol, a natural sugar, have been shown to combat the bacteria associated with dental decay, and some aged cheeses also combat bacteria associated with dental decay. Our BreathRx gum is the only chewing gum I know of that is sweetened with xylitol and has no aspartame.

But you can eat any food without risk of decay—if oral hygiene habits and regular professional care are maintained!

SNACKING

I know it's tough to resist when someone brings in doughnuts or muffins to work, or when you get that "I just have to eat something or I'll die" feeling in the late afternoon. But snacking between meals can be hazardous to your teeth as well as your waistline.

When you eat a complete meal, your body releases lots of saliva, which helps wash food debris away and helps prevent plaque

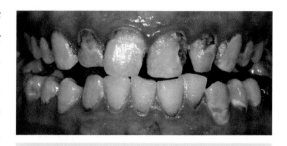

This patient's tooth decay was caused by too much sugar.

buildup; this is not the case with snacking. The other problem is that snack foods often are high in starches and sugars, which break down into destructive acids that eat away at your teeth long after you've finished snacking.

ORAL CANCER

According to the American Dental Association, smoking and drinking alcohol cause an estimated 75 percent of oral cancer in the United States. Don't think that chewing tobacco is safe; it has also been linked to cancer. The easiest solution is to never smoke or use tobacco products!

Sugar hurts your teeth. Tobacco, on the other hand, causes decay, stains your teeth, and, in all likelihood, can kill you. Please do whatever it takes to stop smoking. If not for yourself, at least for those who love you. I lost both grandparents because my grandmother was a chain smoker. Secondhand smoke inhalation can be more deadly than primary inhalation. It killed my nonsmoking grandfather first, and then the same lung cancer killed my grandmother. Sadly, neither of them ever got to meet my beautiful daughters, who are named after them.

In brief, most oral cancers are very aggressive. The American Dental Association says more than seven thousand Americans die every year from oral cancer. As with any cancer, early detection is key, so keep those dental appointments. Your dentist often can spot the signs during a routine checkup. There are also some new diagnostic tests that your dentist can use to detect oral cancer and precancerous areas, with site-specific dyes. If you smoke, live with someone who smokes, or chew tobacco, you should insist on your dentist using one of these tests.

Also, the American Dental Association recommends that you should have your dentist examine any new sore, lump, or discoloration in your mouth that hasn't disappeared within two weeks of discovery. Unless a dentist can identify it definitively, it should be biopsied. Your dentist will normally refer you to an oral surgeon for this. Be sure to follow through! There have been several times when I've insisted on patients' getting a biopsy, even against the recommendations of a physician, and it ended up saving the patients' life.

If you absolutely have to munch on something before your next meal, try foods such as cheese, raw vegetables, plain yogurt, fruits, or nuts. And if you can't brush your teeth after snacking, at least rinse your mouth out with water to help clean away bits of leftover debris.

HEART DISEASE AND DENTAL CARE

Research suggests a strong link between plaque on your teeth and heart disease. The plaque harbors bacteria, and some medical experts believe that when the bacteria enter your bloodstream, they help form blood clots in your coronary arteries, which can cause heart attacks. Or the bacteria in the mouth may weaken your immune system and cause chronic inflammation throughout the entire body—including the coronary arteries. This inflammation in turn contributes to hardening of the arteries.

Another reason to keep your mouth healthy: Recent research has also shown that chronic low-grade oral infections are linked to premature deliveries and lower birth weight in newborns.

So you have more good reasons to practice good oral hygiene and see your dentist regularly.

Keep in mind, all you out there with a sweet tooth, that it's not just cake that causes cavities. There are two types of carbohydrates: simple carbohydrates such as sugar, juice, cake, and candy, and complex carbohydrates such as oatmeal, whole-grain breads, and starchy vegetables. While the latter group has many health benefits, all carbohydrates break down into sugar in your body, and sugar can help cause cavities no matter where it comes from. So from Rice-a-Roni to Rice Krispy Treats, all carbohydrates can be bad for your teeth if you don't brush frequently.

But one of the worst offenders? Candy you suck on for extended periods, and especially breath mints containing sugar.

One of my patients with a beautiful smile had started a new career as a real estate agent. Because she was now in close contact with clients all day long, she was obsessed with having fresh breath. She popped a breath mint beginning, during, and after every meeting, so she was oblivious to the fact that she was bathing her teeth in sugar all day long. Almost one year after she started her new career, she came in for an emergency visit in pain. She ended up with rampant decay, with almost every tooth affected. Her teeth had paid the price of her new mint habit. Her mouth was so riddled with cavities that I had to remove a couple of teeth, perform root canals on several others, and give her a complete set of crowns, veneers, and bridges. In some parts of the country they refer to this as a "full grill." It cost almost fifty thousand dollars for her to avoid dentures.

According to the American Dental Association, tooth decay rates have been declining for many years. However, all dentists are still concerned about the amount of sugar-sweetened sodas and juices that young people are consuming. They have little nutritional value (yes, you should limit your intake of juice, to no more than eight ounces a day) and eventually they'll detrimentally affect your teeth. The sugar in these drinks supplies nourishment for bacteria on the teeth, which in turn produce acid; in conjunction with the acid in most soft drinks, the result can be devastating. If you don't believe me, soak a fork or spoon in a cola drink for twenty-four hours and see what happens. It will eat the metal away!

EATING DISORDERS

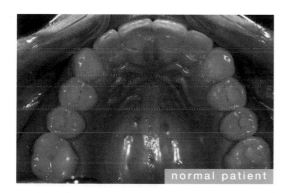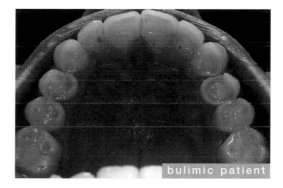

normal patient

bulimic patient

The teeth of the bulimic patient have been damaged by acid. (Normal teeth are shown for comparison.) Notice how much tooth structure is missing due to acid destruction.

I don't need to tell you that eating disorders are unhealthy for a whole host of reasons. But some disorders damage your teeth as well.

Bulimia, binge eating followed by purging or vomiting, brings strong stomach acids to the mouth—acids strong enough to erode enamel over time.

Anorexia, with its excessively restricted eating, isn't much better. Lack of proper minerals and vitamins can destroy the teeth and gums.

I used to treat the members of a famous ballet company and noticed right away that many of the dancers were bulimic. Only a dentist could see it, but there's a classic pattern

THE DENTISTRY DON'TS

Teeth wear down and break. In addition to proper oral hygiene, please consider these additional pointers!

Don't even think about opening a bottle or a wrapper with your teeth. Using your teeth as a can opener or chewing on pens, ice, or popcorn kernels can dull and even crack your teeth. I've probably made enough money fixing teeth cracked on popcorn kernels to buy a luxury car.

Don't even think about showing up to your dentist's office without brushing and flossing. Brush before you come in! The whole office will appreciate it.

Don't even think about letting your child go to bed with a bottle in his or her mouth containing anything but plain water. Milk, formula, and juices can cause what's known as baby bottle tooth decay when they remain on a child's teeth for extended periods.

Don't even think about sucking your thumb. (Yes, some adults suck their thumbs.) It will damage tooth alignment. And pacifiers or bottles for children past the age of two are just as bad.

Don't even think about smoking or chewing tobacco. They not only discolor and weaken your teeth but can lead to gum disease and oral cancer.

Don't even think about going to sleep without brushing and flossing. The plaque will remain on your teeth for an extended period, making you more vulnerable to gingivitis (gum inflammation). Most research shows that if you disrupt or remove plaque and the bacteria it harbors within twenty-four hours, it does not have time to produce enough acid to damage your teeth. At a minimum, once a day is a must!

Don't even think about using OTC tooth-whitening products without your dentist's guidance. These tooth-whitening products are not regulated by the FDA or American Dental Association because they're considered cosmetic, so there's no guarantee they are safe or effective. Plus you may not be a good candidate for whitening, even if they do work.

Don't even think about chewing gum or sucking on lollipops all day—unless they are sugar-free. This includes any substance that will bathe your teeth in sugar for extended periods. When it comes to sugar-free products, I recommend you also avoid aspartame because of all the controversy about possible health risks. The only sugar-free gum or mints I know of sweetened without aspartame are by Discus Dental, in the BreathRx line, and contain xylitol, a natural sweetener that is safe for teeth.

Don't even think about using super-abrasive toothpaste. Sure, it may remove the stain, but it may take part of your tooth along with it.

Don't even think about biting your nails. You can wear your teeth down and chip off the edges.

Don't even think about not wearing your retainer after having braces or other orthodontic treatment. Without the retainer, your teeth will almost certainly return to their original place.

Don't even think about going to a bargain dental center. You get what you pay for, so go to a reputable dentist. See Missy Madrid's story on page 197, and you'll see what I'm talking about.

Don't even think about using someone else's toothbrush. It harbors foreign bacteria that can harm you.

Don't even think about getting your tongue pierced. Tongue piercing can cause excessive drooling; infection, pain, and swelling; chipped teeth; increased saliva flow; and nerve damage. And in many cases, the trauma of the stud or ring gently but repeatedly hitting the lower front teeth can cause the teeth to fall out.

in a bulimic's teeth: severe erosion of the enamel on the inside surface of the teeth. (This differs from the classic erosion you see in people who frequently suck on lemon—they experience erosion on the outside surface of the teeth.) The teeth of bulimics often become so sensitive because of the loss of enamel that it further complicates their eating disorder because it actually becomes painful to eat. Some of the dancers needed full caps or crowns and bridges to replace lost teeth and tooth structure, in some cases costing well over fifty thousand dollars.

dealing
with sensitive teeth

Americans are not as tough as you think. The American Dental Association estimates that approximately 45 million adults complain about sensitive teeth! Have you ever winced after eating ice cream or moaned in pain after taking a sip of coffee? Then you have sensitive teeth. How'd they get that way? Over time some people wear their teeth down with a hard toothbrush or from the acids in foods such as lemons or other citrus fruits, thus exposing dentin, the more sensitive layer beneath the enamel. And as people age, their teeth develop cracks; they may also have receding gums, which exposes the root surface, a very sensitive layer.

Genetically, some people have sensitive teeth even without erosion, cracks, and recession. Everyone is different.

If you have sensitive teeth and you don't want to or cannot give up coffee or ice cream (I haven't touched either in years!), there still is hope. If your dentist diagnoses dentin hypersensitivity, often you can have a coating of composite applied to exposed areas in your teeth. Other products can be brushed on or worn in a tray to bathe your teeth. Many of my patients have found relief by habitually using store-bought toothpastes containing fluoride (which blocks the fluid penetration) and more importantly 5 percent of potassium nitrate (which blocks the nerve). These two ingredients are safe and effective in reducing sensitivity. Allow them at least two weeks to work, and 90 percent of you will be pain free. If you're in the unlucky 10 percent, call your dentist.

bad breath
is bad
news for
relationships

breathe
a little easier

BATTLING BAD BREATH

Chances are you've never been thrown out of anywhere for having bad breath, but I know of a few husbands who have been banished to the couch.

Hundreds of millions of dollars a year are spent on mouthwash. And in most cases, you're gargling your hard-earned money away! The most popular brands of mouthwash do not eliminate bad breath—they only mask it. This is because most of the leading products contain alcohol as the active ingredient. Read the labels—you will be shocked.

The alcohol in these types of mouthwash can actually perpetuate bad breath. You don't need to be a chemist to understand why alcohol doesn't work. Alcohol dries out the soft tissue in your mouth; because saliva is critical to keeping bacteria in check, this actually leads to faster formation of odor-producing bacteria. Also, rinses containing alcohol have been shown to cause uncomfortable irritation in users; they can also alter oral tissues, which further contributes to malodor. So alcohol-based mouthwashes are actually counterproductive! Everybody should avoid mouthwashes with alcohol, especially children, diabetics, recovering alcoholics, and pregnant mothers. (Yes, there are some alcohol-free mouthwashes out there—including one made by Discus Dental; see page 151.)

Millions are also spent on "breath-freshening" chewing gums and mints. Unfortunately, these also only mask odors. They don't get rid of them.

what causes bad breath?

What is bad breath, anyway? It's the result of odor-causing bacteria that create waste materials in the mouth. Food particles get trapped in the creases and grooves and especially on the fissures of the tongue, and become nutrition for bacteria. And when these bacteria feed, they release gaseous waste products that cause foul-smelling odors known as volatile sulfur compounds (VSCs). The odor of these gases is similar to that of rotten eggs. You probably know what that smells like!

We all have bad breath sometimes. There are two types of bad breath:

Transitory bad breath. This is short lasting and usually comes from eating foods such as garlic or onions. It can also be just a case of morning breath. As we sleep, saliva production is decreased and this allows bacteria to proliferate. The result is morning breath.

Chronic bad breath. This is the long-lasting type that makes people wince. I like to refer to this as the "long-term relationship killer" and this is also called halitosis.

Here are the most common factors that can lead to both types of bad breath:

Food particles. If you don't remove all the tiny bits of food from your mouth and between your teeth through proper brushing and flossing, bad breath can result. Also if you have gingivitis or periodontal disease, you will harbor much more bacteria than usual.

Bacteria. If you don't scrape your tongue properly, the film of bacteria in all the little crevices of your tongue can produce an unpleasant odor. Up to 90 percent of oral bad odor originates at the back of your tongue. In addition to the normal accumulation of bacteria found here, millions of people suffer from post-nasal drip, sometimes without being aware of it. The mucus that drips down onto the back of the tongue is broken down by your mouth's bacteria, causing even more odor.

BAD BREATH CONTROL PACKAGE

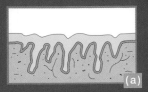 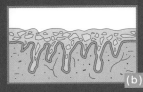 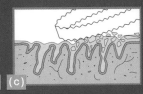 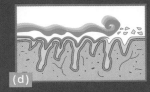

(a) (b) (c) (d)

Here's how the BreathRx breath control system works: (a) The deep pockets of the tongue harbor debris, bacteria, and plaque. (b) ZYTEX penetrates and loosens the odor-causing bacteria. (c) The tongue scraper lifts and removes debris and bacteria. (d) The antibacterial mouth rinse flushes the loosened particles and leaves ZYTEX to continue working.

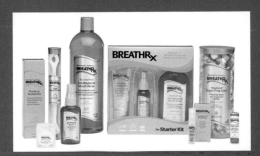

BreathRx product line.

Discus Dental offers an excellent breath control system called BreathRx. It contains mouthwash, toothpaste, floss, a tongue scraper (most bad breath originates on the tongue), tongue scraping spray, mints, and gum. BreathRx mouthwash and all the other products are alcohol free and eliminate bad breath, rather than just masking it. Unlike most odor-fighting and oral care products on the market today, they actually attack the cause of bad breath.

A proprietary ingredient in all BreathRx products called ZYTEX, along with other ingredients, works with a one-two punch to eliminate bad breath. The combination of these products first kills the odor-causing bacteria, then neutralizes the gas they produce. The system's three-step approach takes just a few minutes.

1. **Brush and floss.** The BreathRx toothpaste attacks those stubborn volatile sulfur compounds with ZYTEX and a complex of potent ingredients. But that's not all. BreathRx toothpaste also contains fluoride for everyday use, and BreathRx floss is impregnated with ZYTEX for maximum bacterial kill.

2. **Scrape.** The BreathRx tongue spray coats the surface of the tongue and seeps into the fissures to kill and loosen bacteria. Simply use the BreathRx tongue scraper to scrape away those bacteria. Remember that a toothbrush only spreads the debris around—use a tongue scraper to sweep it out!

3. **Rinse.** BreathRx mouth rinse has a pleasant mint flavor and because it contains no alcohol, it tastes less medicinal than most mouthwashes. Studies show that using this rinse over time actually improves your breath with a cumulative effect. No other antibacterial mouth rinse can make this claim. Studies also show that BreathRx outperforms the leading alcohol-containing mouthwashes.

Throughout the day, you can refresh your breath with the spray, mints, or the Halosphere gum (my favorite). You can purchase this breath-control package at www.BreathRx.com, your dentist's office, or almost any drugstore.

Dry mouth. Also called xerostomia (pronounced *zero-stow-me-uh*), dry mouth results from a lack of saliva because of age, medication, or loss of saliva glands from surgery or radiation therapy. Aside from causing bad breath, it can lead to tooth decay and gum disease because saliva flow helps clean and shield the mouth and teeth. Over-the-counter artificial saliva replacements, a manmade version of what your mouth normally produces, help some patients. However, others find that chewing sugar-free gum or having sugar-free candy helps prevent the mouth from drying out by increasing saliva production.

Medicine. Hundreds of medications, especially for diabetes, can cause dry mouth. As mentioned, you can buy artificial saliva that may help keep your mouth lubricated. But sugar-free gum or candy may also stimulate saliva flow.

Dieting. When you diet, your body goes into survival mode called ketosis. Stomach fluids called ketones are produced when you fast or diet, giving off an odor that is not quite the same as the usual bad breath smell, which results from just bacteria. I smell this odor on all my *Extreme Makeover* patients as the pounds melt away. It is distinct, pungent, and unavoidable under many diets.

Smoking. Smoking is also a major culprit because it dries out your mouth and leaves a foul-smelling residue. Also, you don't need a dentist to tell you that smoking causes a lot more problems than just bad breath.

Alcohol. Alcohol—whether you are drinking it or using an alcohol-containing mouth rinse—ruins your breath for reasons I've discussed. Alcohol dries out your mouth and prevents saliva from keeping bacteria in check.

Illness. A very small percentage of bad breath offenders are suffering from a serious sickness, such as liver problems, cancer, or tonsillitis. When all else fails to indicate a cause for bad breath, see your medical doctor.

why you need to fix the problem

Bad breath is bad news for relationships. I know of a woman, let's call her Lucy, a smart, sassy lawyer who started seeing a really nice guy. Things were looking pretty good. Unfortunately, they weren't smelling too good.

The guy was perfect in every way except for his breath. He was attractive and cultured and even cooked for her. Only problem: She couldn't stand his breath.

Lucy said that when they kissed it tasted like the inside of a tuna can. Wait, it gets worse: a tuna can that's been sitting in the trash for a couple of days!

Okay, maybe she was exaggerating, but the sad truth was Lucy couldn't stand to kiss him. And she wanted to kiss him. She said she felt really superficial that his breath bothered her so much, but it was becoming a deal-breaker.

Unfortunately, having bad breath is not like having acne. You can't see it. Most people don't even know they have it. Others can detect it, but it's hard to detect on your own. And most people won't tell you when you have it.

Well, Lucy's boyfriend didn't know he had it, and when Lucy delicately revealed it to him he immediately became defensive and embarrassed. And that was the end of that. He chose to stop seeing her rather than deal with the humiliating situation. By the way, Lucy has since moved on to another guy who, she says, has wonderfully fresh breath.

Bad breath can also wreak havoc in the office. One of my patients works with a guy, let's call him Brad, who had such bad breath that his coworkers actually complained. It became a human resources issue! This man's breath was so horrible, his colleagues called his work area "the danger zone." It smelled like a dead body.

His coworkers were too uncomfortable to say anything to him, but the human resources director was not. Brad was told that his breath was creating an uncomfortable work environment and he needed to do something about it ASAP. Once Brad started using the BreathRx system (see page 151), the situation was immediately resolved.

Bad breath affects millions. Unfortunately, most of those who have it don't even know it!

how do I know
if I have bad breath?

See, this is where having good friends comes in handy. Remember that friend who always tells you the truth? Well, that's the friend you want to call and ask if you have bad breath because most people won't say a thing—to your face, anyway!

If you don't have friends like that, some scientists suggest a test you can try: Lick your wrist (from as far back on the tongue as possible because that's where the nastiest bacteria live), let your saliva dry for a few seconds, and then take a whiff. Not very scientific, I know, and I can't vouch for its effectiveness.

For a while, dentists tried using a halitometer, a sulfide monitor that gauges the gases in your breath to test for bad breath. Unfortunately, this device is not very accurate, and I don't recommend it.

Of the hundreds of bacteria varieties that call your mouth home, some are especially putrid. The oral bacteria that feed off food particles in your mouth produce hydrogen sulfide, which smells like, you got it, rotten eggs.

With odors like that, it's no wonder millions suffer from halitophobia, a fear of hav-

MORNING BREATH

Bedhead, bloodshot eyes, and morning breath. All good reasons to pull the covers over your head and stay in bed all day. We all have to face the world every day but some of us are fortunate enough to face someone we love in the morning when we rise and shine. As glad as that someone may be to see us, no one welcomes morning breath.

Brush and floss carefully before bed so food particles don't get the chance to break down overnight and make your morning breath even worse. Keep a glass of water by the bed and have some before going to bed, and as soon as you wake up take another big swig because bad breath is caused, in part, by dry mouth.

If your morning breath doesn't go away after brushing your teeth, well, your morning breath has been upgraded to chronic bad breath. And no one wants bad breath that lasts all day long. If that's the case, try the BreathRx system or our bad breath fixes (see pages 151 and 155). Or go see your dentist about treating halitosis.

ing halitosis. As far as phobias go, in my opinion, this one's not that bad. But I say don't fear it, change it.

how to fix bad breath

Having bad breath isn't like having body odor. You can't just take a shower and change your clothes and it goes away. It requires diligent dental care and a change in lifestyle. But you can do it. Here are some tips on how to combat bad breath.

Practice regular dental hygiene. Brush your teeth at least twice a day, preferably three times, and floss too! And don't forget to scrape that tongue because that's where most of the bacteria that cause bad breath live. (Remember, it's important to scrape the tongue, not brush it; see page 134.)

Drink plenty of water. Throw back at least eight glasses of water a day (you can't make saliva if you are not well hydrated) and cut down on the coffee, which not only gives you "coffee breath" but stains your teeth as well.

Change your diet. Some foods are tougher for your body to break down than others. Beans, onions, and garlic produce gases that cause bad breath. Eat more fresh fruits and veggies. Remember, carrots and apples naturally help to clean your teeth and your breath, and chewing on fresh mint also does wonders—but of course these are no substitutes for regular brushing and flossing.

Chew gum (sugarless of course). Chewing gum creates saliva, which creates a moist mouth, usually resulting in better breath than a dry mouth. But remember, breath-freshening gum only helps to refresh bad breath. It doesn't cure it! (And I recommend avoiding products with aspartame for health reasons.)

Change your mouthwash. Select an alcohol-free mouthwash by reading the labels.

it's never too late to begin your life again

8

now spit!

TALES FROM THE CHAIR

In my Beverly Hills practice, I create Billion Dollar Smiles for many, many million-aires and A-listers from Hollywood and around the world. I'm sharing some of their stories with you here because they can offer you insights into your own smile makeover.

Sometimes it's the most macho athletes that are reduced to the biggest wimps in a dental office. That's okay. I treat all my patients with special care. If anyone needs a little extra attention, my staff and I are more than happy to oblige.

Ozzy Osbourne

Take the one and only Ozzy Osbourne. He not only gets extra attention, he gets extra anesthesia! I've been the Osbourne family dentist for many years now. I knew, well before MTV got wind of it, that they were a loving, caring, loud, wild family. Ozzy says that Sharon definitely wears the pants, but Ozzy wears the crown—he is the king of his domain. His family likes to joke with him, and

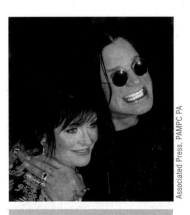

Ozzy and Sharon
Osbourne

MY DATE WITH A DESPERATE HOUSEWIFE

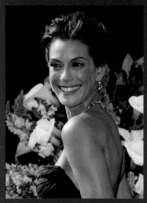

Teri Hatcher

Jay Leno is famous for a lot of things. He has his own network show, he collects cars, and he has a famous profile. What you might not know about Jay is that he's also a matchmaker! Jay asked his guest Teri Hatcher, the hottest bachelorette on the block and a star of the television show *Desperate Housewives*, if she was dating anyone. When she said no, he asked if she had a crush on anyone on TV. Blushing, Teri admitted she wanted to meet "that dentist on *Extreme Makeover*." Jay went in for the kill and set us up—on national television.

Here's how it happened: I was speaking at a dental convention in Sweden when Jay's producer called me and informed me that one of their guests wanted to go out with me. When I asked who, she replied, "Teri Hatcher." I thought she was kidding, and I was just about to hang up when she convinced me that this was no joke. She asked if I was up for a setup, and being single at the time, I did not hesitate to say yes. My conversation with the producer had been taped, and it aired on the show as Teri sat on Jay's couch, embarrassed and blushing. I was on top of the world! I was single and had just told a friend that I thought Teri was attractive and wondered if I would ever meet her.

Teri told Jay she was worried that if things didn't work out with me I wouldn't work on her teeth. As if there isn't enough pressure on a first date!

Teri asked Jay, "Do you really want to date somebody who's been looking at the inside of your mouth for five hours?" Without missing a beat, Jay said, "Well, he'll probably do that anyway!" The audience had a good laugh.

Being my persistent and (I hope!) charming self, I sent Teri flowers and a box of chocolates before our date with a note that said, "Dear Teri, in case you are getting cold feet about our first date, please eat this box of chocolates so I can at least see you when you need to get your cavities filled." I'm not sure if she ate the candy, but she showed up and we had a wonderful time. We quickly found out we had a lot in common. We were both divorced, fiercely dedicated single parents balancing demanding careers and lives in the ABC-Disney family. All right, Teri was a mega-star and I was just "that dentist." But you get the idea. We went only on one date, but Teri invited me to her fortieth birthday party, which was coming up soon. The party was like a real-life episode of *Desperate Housewives.* All of Wisteria Lane was there, and I ended up hanging out with a couple of other housewives, the lovely Eva Longoria and Marcia Cross.

Teri is a smart, sexy woman and a great actress with a Billion Dollar Smile to boot. I wish her the best. And yes, I will still work on her smile.

One lesson I learned from my date with Teri is that she is a walking, talking example of a comeback. She proves that it's never too late to begin your life again. When Teri won the Golden Globe for *Desperate Housewives*, she spoke eloquently and honestly about being, in her words, a "has-been" who was given a second chance. You might feel like that too some days. We all do. But I firmly believe that sometimes a new smile can change all that and give you that second chance you're looking for.

he is a great sport with a great sense of humor. Rest assured, Daddy is adored by his lovely wife, Sharon, and the kids. I was honored to attend the renewal of their marriage vows on Sharon's fiftieth birthday, and it was one of the most touching ceremonies I have ever seen.

In my dental practice we have low, medium, and high settings for laughing gas. But when Ozzy comes in, we have to turn it to the "Ozzy" setting. The maximum amount of gas usually isn't enough!

You may have watched Ozzy come into my office on an MTV episode of *The Osbournes*. The cameras followed Ozzy into my office for a visit. Now, it's no secret that my rock 'n' roll patients had a lot of fun in the '70s and '80s. Perhaps as a result, Ozzy seems to have quite a resistance to gas. Because when we turn on the laughing gas (nitrous oxide), he barely feels a thing.

We have to keep turning it up well past what is usually effective on non–rock star icons. As the MTV cameras rolled, Ozzy kept saying he didn't feel anything, so we turned it up. Again, he mumbled something about not feeling anything. So we cranked the gas as far as it goes—to what we call "Ozzy level." Finally that got him happy.

We heard him mumble "nitrous" a few times when he was under. But when we were finished, he botched the rinse. He kept hitting the cup against his head, not his mouth. We try not to laugh at our patients, but that was pretty funny—even Ozzy got a kick out of it.

He laughs about it too. That's what makes him such a great guy—although he doesn't take himself or the world too seriously, he's a wonderful, warm human being. There was a time in my life when I was going through relationship problems and when Ozzy saw how hard it was on me, he took time out of his busy schedule to call me and offer a shoulder to lean on. He is a real gentleman with a huge heart, and it has been a pleasure and honor to take care of him and his family for the past decade and a half. If you ask Ozzy, he always gives all the credit to Sharon—who really is amazing—but he's just as amazing in his own right.

Esther Williams

Esther Williams is Hollywood royalty, a million dollar mermaid with a Billion Dollar Smile. The bathing beauty was an MGM mega-star who appeared in dozens of films:

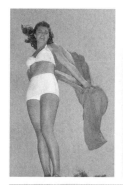
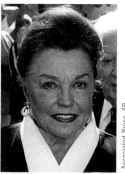

Associated Press, AP

Esther Williams

THE SMILE THAT BROUGHT LOVE INTO MY LIFE

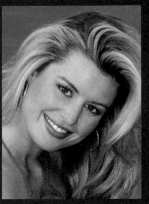

Jennifer Murphy

Smiles have played such a large part in my life, both personally and professionally, from my experience as a small child losing my teeth to my becoming a dentist. And it was a smile that brought love into my life when I least expected it.

In 2004 I was hoping to judge the Miss USA pageant at the Kodak Theater in Hollywood, home of the Academy Awards. But a few weeks before the pageant, I was told that the network needed more NBC actors, not an ABC dentist, to judge the competition. However, NBC arranged for me to attend as a spectator.

Within the first ten minutes of the show, when all of the contestants make their initial pass on the stage, I was immediately drawn to the most beautiful woman on the stage by her flawless figure—and of course her smile. The second I saw Jennifer Murphy, Miss Oregon 2004, I knew that her Billion Dollar Smile and beautiful, sexy yet natural look would make her a perfect spokesperson for Discus Dental, my dental company. I shared this thought with my friends and just by chance, Carol Lukens, the director for Miss Oregon, was sitting right behind me and overheard my comment. She put me in touch with Jennifer, but because of production delays we didn't shoot the commercials for another year. So almost exactly one year after first seeing Jennifer, I phoned her and flew her down to L.A. to audition.

As I expected, everyone at Discus Dental fell in love with her and thought she would be great for our company image. So the next day I called her to tell her that we would use her for the next campaign, and to my surprise she was flustered. When I asked her what was wrong, she said that she had been so inspired by me, my dental office, and Discus Dental that she had returned home and done something she had wanted to do for a long time. She was ready to drive down to San Diego to audition for Donald Trump's *The Apprentice*. I told her that if she made that fourteen-hour drive she would be too tired to do well in the audition, and I asked her how far she was from the closest airport. I have tons of air miles from all the traveling I do for my lectures, so I offered to get her a ticket.

Apparently the casting people for the show also loved her—except for Mark Burnett, who thought Jennifer was too beautiful to be taken seriously. That is when The Donald stepped in. The *New York Times* quotes him as saying, "Number one, she's smart. Number two, she's beautiful. Congratulations, she's on the show."

Even though Jennifer got fired before the end of the season, Mr. Trump offered her a job at the conclusion of the season. So in essence she won a spot as his apprentice, and under normal circumstances she would have taken the job. But something unexpected happened along the way. I out-trumped Trump! Jennifer couldn't accept the job, which was in New York, because I had proposed to her and we wanted to continue to live in L.A.

Originally I had fallen in love with her smile, and after getting to know her I fell head over heels for her. She is an amazing woman, as loving and sweet as she is beautiful. While some cast members on *The Apprentice* are mean and cutthroat, she proved you can get what you want with a smile. Even a dentist!

in her trademark underwater spectaculars featuring synchronized swimming, and in other movies in which she starred as a walking, talking mortal on dry land.

Esther Williams was the first celebrity patient I ever worked on in my private practice. I had just opened my own practice in the Beverly Hills area when she walked in for a consultation. She said, "Dr. Dorfman, I know a lot of people think that my career is slowing down, but I'm still being photographed all the time and I want to have that Esther Williams smile I was famous for back again."

I said, "Esther, you bring me a studio photo of you with that famous smile, and I promise you I'll give you back that smile." She looked at me and said, "Dr. Dorfman, with all due respect, are you old enough to be doing this?"

I replied, "Esther, sit back, relax, and I promise to take good care of you." And through the magic of cosmetic dentistry, I rejuvenated her smile. She's been a loyal patient ever since.

As we became close personal friends, my admiration for Esther grew. I once teased her, saying, "Esther, if you were fifty years younger, I'd want to marry you." Without skipping a beat, she replied, "You'd be smart to, because I've made a lot of money in my lifetime."

Esther jokingly told me in front of her personal assistant, Debbie, that Debbie has made the commitment to stay with her for the rest of her life. Esther looked at me with that twinkle in her eye and said, "Dr. Dorfman, you're on the same plan."

The pleasure is mine, Esther.

Jessica Simpson

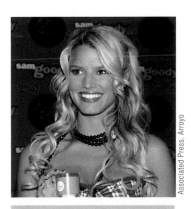

Jessica Simpson

You may have seen Jessica Simpson bravely endure her dental drama on her MTV reality show *The Newlyweds*. I had been begging the sweet and adorable star for two years to let me fill a cavity, but she kept so busy it never happened. Finally it got so bad that she visited my office during her show, moaning and complaining of a toothache. She had told me earlier that she'd never had a root canal, but I knew immediately that she needed one now. So here's how I broke the news to her. I said, "Jessica, I have good news and bad news. The bad news is that you definitely need a root canal. The good news is that I get to tell all my friends that I was your first—root canal, that is!"

The next time she came in, I made her a badge that said in big letters "I was Jessica Simpson's first" and then in small letters "root canal." At least I was first at something in her life.

On Jessica's first visit I told her she had to floss more, and she said she hated flossing with a passion. Do the math! That's why she needed a root canal.

As the camera rolled, she sat in my chair saying, "I hate this." I told her she had waited way too long on this one, and she admitted her guilt. But to her credit, she is one of the busiest celebs out there and one of the most photographed women in the world.

I told her to try to lay off the sugar. On the way out of the office, she grabbed a handful of my sugar-free gumballs from the jar on the receptionist's desk. As far as I know she listened to me, at least until she got to the elevator—because she was filmed that far!

Sergeant Aaron Wintterle

Sergeant Aaron J. Wintterle is a celebrity of another sort: an American hero. He was a member of a scout sniper platoon with the 1st Marine Division, 7th regiment, 3rd Battalion, in Iraq when he came under attack and was nearly killed.

This young marine received a Purple Heart from military officials, but I gave him a brand-new smile. The scout sniper and his unit were guarding a road intersection when

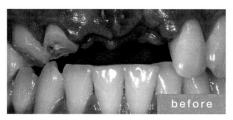

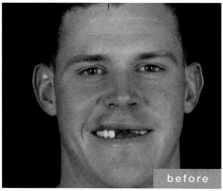

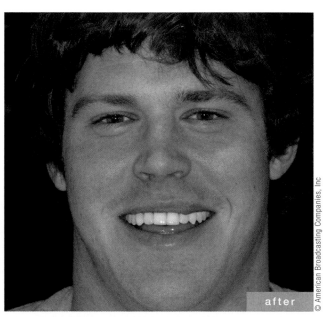

Cosmetic dentistry restored Sergeant Wintterle's smile through implants and veneers.

they were ambushed. He took shrapnel to the teeth and not only lost his teeth, but also nearly lost his life.

There were five suicide bombers trying to bring his unit down. When he got hit, he was knocked out for a few seconds and woke up thinking he was going to die. When he realized he might actually survive, he crawled under cover and one of his buddies held a T-shirt to his face to stop the bleeding. A few minutes later, and still under heavy fire, they threw him in a truck and took him to a medic at the American checkpoint.

Sergeant Wintterle says that while he believes in fighting for his country, it was then that he understood the absurdity of war. The very Iraqis who had shot at him were being treated on the cots right next to him.

His lip was split open, two front teeth were completely blown out, and his two remaining front teeth were broken in half. He almost lost his tongue and suffered bone damage to his jaw. Sergeant Wintterle knows he was lucky to be alive.

One of my patients, Owen McKibben, a *Men's Health* cover and fitness model, saw Sergeant Wintterle on CNN and told me what had happened. I thought, "What a tragedy for such a young guy to spend the rest of his life crippled with a broken smile." I told my office manager to phone the CNN network and ask them to have Sergeant Wintterle contact me if he wanted a smile makeover. I felt the least I could do for a man who nearly gave his life for our country was to pay him back with a few teeth. Needless to say, I didn't charge him for the procedures, nor did Dr. Ari Rosenblatt, the Beverly Hills periodontist and implant doctor.

We gave Sergeant Wintterle two implants for the teeth that were blown out and two porcelain veneers for the broken teeth next to them. His smile was as good as new.

Sergeant Wintterle loves his new smile almost as much as his old one. He says, "You can't replace real teeth but they're pretty close." He now manages a lumberyard in Missouri and studies criminal justice at night at a local university. He claims that his new smile has changed his life and has given him the second chance he needed. I'm proud that I was able to help this young man adjust to his new life.

Sergeant Wintterle says that even though he is physically home now, he is not necessarily home in spirit. His thoughts and prayers are very much with his buddies back in Iraq.

take a
good look
at your
dentist's
smile

9

this won't hurt a bit

HOW TO HAVE
A GREAT RELATIONSHIP
WITH A GREAT DENTIST

First let's define our terms. What is a good dentist?

First and foremost, he or she is a qualified person with whom you feel comfortable. It doesn't matter how many degrees this dentist has. If you don't feel physically and emotionally comfortable, it won't be a good experience.

It's widely believed that dentist loyalty is one of the highest of all professions. Many people will change their physician, their broker, their accountant, their hairdresser, their trainer, and even their clergyman before they change their dentist.

Second, you should check out educational background. It's pretty safe to say that dentists who graduated from a reputable dental school and received a good dental education should at least know their stuff. Any dental school in the United States or Canada will do—you can find lists at www.ada.org (American Dental Association) or www.adea.org (American Dental Education Association). International ones may not fit the bill.

Third, find out how much continuing education they have taken. Look at the certificates on the wall and ask if you don't see any. Staying up to date on this ever-changing field is crucial. I've been practicing dentistry for more than twenty years, and 99 percent of what I do today I didn't learn in dental school. Porcelain veneers didn't even *exist* before the mid-eighties. I learned new technology along the way. Make sure your dentist is up-to-date. Find out if your dentist is a member of any dental academies.

Word of mouth, pun intended, will help you find a quality dental professional. Ask your friends and ask your physicians. Another health-care provider will usually know who's good and who's not so good.

Try reaching out to the AACD (American Academy of Cosmetic Dentistry). It recommends only accredited members, those who've gone through a series of rigorous tests. For help finding a cosmetic dentist, the AACD online referral system is at www.aacd.com and the toll-free number is 1-800-543-9220. For orthodontists, contact the American Association of Orthodontists at www.braces.org or call 1-800-STRAIGHT.

You can also go online and see if the dentist you are considering has ever been sued for malpractice. (Just search for the dentist's name and the word "malpractice.") If a dentist—or any medical professional—has multiple suits filed, I'd be leery.

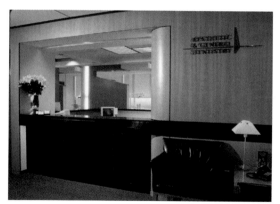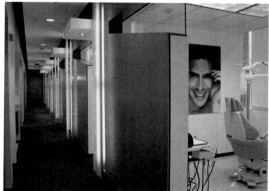

The reception area and hallway of my office.

You should also be leery if your dentist's office isn't clean, modern, and state-of-the-art. If the carpets are dirty and the equipment is taped together with duct tape or looks like something from a 1950s science fiction movie, you can probably assume that dentist isn't practicing cutting-edge dentistry.

Once you've selected a dentist that you trust and place your mouth in his or her care, it's important that you communicate your cosmetic desires as clearly and succinctly as possible. If you're the type of person who puts 100 percent faith in your dentist's hands and just want him or her to make the selections as far as shape, size, color, and style of your teeth, that's fine. However, it has been my experience—which may be skewed because of where I practice, in Beverly Hills—that most patients want to have a lot of input. I think you *should* have something to say about it. After all, you're the one who is going to wear the smile, not the dentist.

things to check out

Some criteria to sink your teeth into when searching for a new dentist:

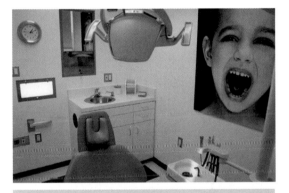
The examinatioin room in my office.

> Every dental office should sterilize instruments in accordance with OSHA (Occupational Safety and Health Administration) guidelines. Ask your dentist if you're not sure. A dentist should not be offended by this question.

> Every person working on you should wear masks, gloves, and eye protection, to protect themselves and you as well.

> Your dentist's employees should be friendly and competent. Do they have attractive smiles? Chances are that dentist is responsible for their smiles.

> Take a good look at your dentist's smile. You have to practice what you preach. Would you go to an overweight trainer? My smile is like my business card.

> Your dentist should be warm, friendly, and open to suggestions and discussion. Your new smile should be a collaborative effort.

Always ask how much cosmetic dentistry the dentist does. Just a few cases a year is not a lot of experience. Ask to see "before and after" pictures of smiles this dentist created.

Be aware that a lot of dentists use stock photos, representative photos that are not of their patients, so it's critical you ask if it's their work shown in the photos. I actually sold some of my "before and after" smiles to a company years ago. One of my patients who had been smile shopping said she had seen one of my signature smiles in another dentist's office—and the dentist claimed *he* had performed the dental work in the picture.

Once you establish a relationship with your dentist and you need a specialist such as an oral surgeon, periodontist (gum specialist), or endodontist (root canal specialist), ask your general or cosmetic dentist for a recommendation or referral. To receive the best care, it's important that both dentists communicate and are on the same page. Procedures such as implants or gum surgery are a group effort: The specialist and the general or cosmetic dentist have to work together.

Cosmetic dentistry is *not* an American Dental Association board–recognized specialty. So a big red flag should go up if your new dentist claims to "specialize in cosmetic dentistry." In fact, it is a violation of the dentists' code of ethics to even make such a statement.

If you go to a specialist, be advised that most dentists don't double up on specialties. In other words, you don't want a root canal specialist recontouring your smile. And if you have doubts about dental treatment, always get a second opinion. As with any medical procedure, it's always helpful to hear what another professional has to say.

fear of dentists: dentophobia

Dentophobia, or fear of dentists, is an irrational fear that plagues rational people. Even I can understand why some people might find it a little uncomfortable to have strangers hovering over their faces and sticking their hands (never mind their drills!) in their mouths. But dentophobia goes beyond this normal discomfort. It's a fear that paralyzes millions. It's much more common than a lot of dentists would like to admit. We prefer to think that our patients, even the nervous ones, come in because they love us, not because they have to!

I've had patients so afraid of dentists, they come in only when the pain is so bad they can barely speak. And these are relatively healthy people who otherwise take care of themselves and lead productive lives. But when it comes to the dentist, they'd almost rather endure the toothaches than sit in the chair.

The chair, by the way, is not the electric chair. Many dentists go out of their way to make the dental experience as comfortable and scare-free as possible. But comfort isn't going to cure your fears.

Why are people afraid of dentists? Most of the dentists I know are wonderful, caring human beings. The dental community believes there are many possible reasons:

> A childhood trauma at the dentist you never really got over
> A feeling of shame or fear of being blamed for your bad teeth or dental problems
> Fear of pain
> Fear of the unknown
> Fear of needles
> Dental horror stories you may have heard—I won't repeat any because that'll only make you more nervous!
> Fear of losing control

There are many ways to combat dentophobia.

Find a dentist you trust. This is paramount. This is where word of mouth comes into play. Ask your most demanding, high-maintenance friends whom they see. (Finally, they're good for something!) A good dentist will listen to your concerns and not dismiss them.

Explain your fears. Your dentist and assistants can help if you explain your fears (no matter how irrational) to them. Trust me, they don't want you having a panic attack any more than you do. You can agree on a signal if you need them to pause during a procedure.

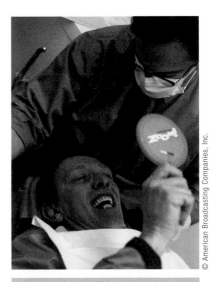

© American Broadcasting Companies, Inc.

It is important to find a dentist you can trust.

Ask questions. Your dentist needs to lend a hand in the effort to reassure you and should discuss whatever procedures are being done. You should feel comfortable asking any and all questions you have about the procedure. Having this knowledge is empowering; it will help dispel the fear of the unknown.

Find a soothing place to go. Create a calming scenario in your mind. Picture yourself lying on a hammock by the beach or relaxing by the fireplace at your parents' house. If thinking about your parents causes even more anxiety, then how about sitting by a stream in the woods? All of us have a "safe" place we can think of. If you go there in your mind, you'll be surprised how calming that can be.

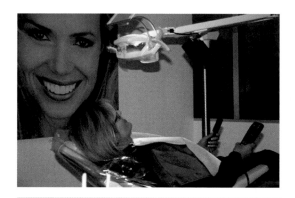

A patient relaxes during her dental visit with safety glasses, a blanket, a TV remote, and a remote for a back-massage unit.

Distract yourself. Listen to music or books on tape with headphones. You could also distract yourself by watching TV or using virtual reality glasses that let you watch and listen to videos as your mouth is being worked on. Many dentists today can supply these.

Use calming techniques. Yoga provides good relaxation breathing techniques that combat anxiety. When you're at the dentist, remember to breathe deeply and slowly. If you can control your breathing, you'll be amazed how well you can control your anxiety levels.

Have a hand to hold. Sometimes having a friend or family member come along to your appointment can help assuage your fears. Having someone you love hold your hand during a procedure can provide an enormous amount of comfort and moral support. Of course, your dentist will have to determine if having another person in the room is appropriate for whatever procedure you're having done.

Remember that fear is something we learn, and it is a behavior that can be unlearned. Also realize that dentophobia can be a self-fulfilling prophecy: If you put off a dental visit because of fear, and if you are in great pain or need extensive invasive procedures by the time you do drag yourself into the office, you're reinforcing your concept of the dental office as a horrible place.

Keep in mind that you are a paying customer and you have the right to make sure your needs are met in your dentist's office. If you need some special attention, don't hesitate to ask. If your dentist hesitates to give you special care, look for a dentist who will. They are out there. (If all else fails, book an appointment with me!)

As a second to last resort, mild sedatives recommended by your dentist could ease your mind. Options include nitrous oxide or oral tranquilizers. As a last resort, you may need general anesthesia. (See Chapter 4 for more information.)

And never be afraid or ashamed to admit you are afraid and you need help.

you,
too, can
reinvent
yourself

10

making dreams
come true

DENTAL MAKEOVER MIRACLES

People have made a big deal over the doctors who appear on *Extreme Makeover*. But the real heroes are the patients themselves. They are incredibly brave, exposing their vulnerabilities and sharing their dreams and desires on national television. Not to mention the fact that they literally expose themselves by posing in their underwear for the world to see all their flaws.

On television, you get to see what the *Extreme Makeover* candidates look like only at their "reveal" parties—you don't really get to know these people or see how these changes affect their lives after the show is over. I caught up with some of my very special and most challenging patients from the show. As they talked about how their new smiles had changed their lives, I noticed a reoccurring theme: Nearly all of them spoke about second chances.

Life doesn't generally give anyone a second chance at anything, but these lucky souls have experienced the extraordinary opportunity to reinvent themselves (with a little help) from their smiles to their souls.

You, too, can reinvent yourself—whether by improving your smile, getting fit, finding a new job, or changing your outlook on life. I hope these stories will inspire you!

a rapper's rap: the Jeff Oliphant story

Jeff Oliphant's story is a testament to how family can bond together and triumph over adversity.

BEFORE THE MAKEOVER

Jeff is an aspiring rap artist with a heart of gold. Unfortunately, he was born with a cleft palate (a split in the roof of the mouth that can cause many other problems). Jeff had worn braces since the sixth grade, but his teeth weren't getting any better. And then his family couldn't afford to continue his orthodontic treatment, so his dental problem eventually devolved into a dental crisis without a foreseeable solution—before *Extreme Makeover*.

In addition to the problems Jeff had with the appearance of his smile, the cleft gave him a severe speech defect. Imagine trying to talk with a hole going from the roof of your mouth into your sinuses.

I had to use every trick in the book to tackle Jeff's dental dilemma. Among other problems, I needed to fill a big gap. Normally, with a bridge you hook the artificial teeth to other surrounding teeth. But Jeff's teeth were loose because of the abnormal bone support in the cleft area, so they were not strong enough to support a conventional bridge. I contemplated removing his two front teeth and giving him a removable appliance to make his smile work, but vetoed that plan because I wanted him to keep his teeth. Finally, I figured out a way to keep his two front teeth and make a permanent bridge in addition to porcelain veneers for beautiful teeth.

But a beautiful smile is more than just beautiful teeth—it also involves the lips. Fixing a cleft lip and palate is especially delicate and time-consuming. Often multiple procedures are necessary to get it right. In fact, as a child Jeff had endured several surgeries that failed to do the job.

HOW WE FIXED JEFF'S SMILE

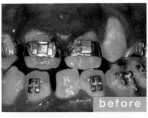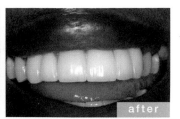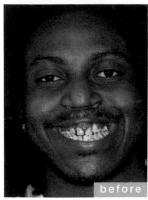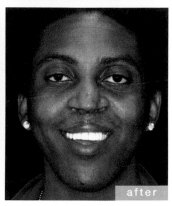

Jeff Oliphant's Extreme Makeover included lip repositioning, ZOOM! whitening, porcelain veneers, crowns, and permanent bridges.

I was not about to give up on Jeff. This case required a team effort, so I worked in tandem with a plastic surgeon. We performed a scar revision and lip repositioning, which normally tacks the lip down to hide a gummy smile. In this instance, we used the procedure to hide the cleft palate. We also took off his braces and treated his teeth with ZOOM! in-office whitening, getting them fifteen shades whiter—from brown to white. Jeff also received two permanent bridges and eleven porcelain veneers and crowns to make his smile more even.

After all the work was complete, Jeff's speech improved dramatically. Don't forget, I treat Ozzy Osbourne, so I'm pretty good at understanding difficult-to-understand speech patterns, but now everyone else could understand him too.

Jeff says his life has changed just as dramatically. Before, he didn't get many looks, at least not positive looks. Now people are more open. All he has to do is flash his new bright smile and people instantly feel like he is approachable. Now, he can walk into a room and just be Jeff, not that guy with the cleft palate.

Jeff's smile makeover has had an amazing effect on not only him, but also his entire family. There were tears of joy at Jeff's reveal. His family's reaction to his new smile was, "We did it! We made it!" It was the miracle they had all been praying for.

According to Jeff, people who've seen him on the show stop him in airports and restaurants and ask if they can hug him. But it is the people he knows best whose reactions mean the most to him. He says, "The magic to me was seeing people I knew. It was like everyone was seeing me for the first time. You know how they say you can never give a second first impression—well, you can." Jeff is certainly proof of that.

Jeff was particularly grateful to me for his new smile. Every other dentist who looked at him was afraid to treat him, but he could tell how excited I was by the challenge. In fact, he said, "I've never seen anyone who likes teeth as much as Dr. Dorfman."

Jeff says that his family always pictured him with a normal, healthy smile. So reality TV helped his family catch up with the reality of their hearts and minds.

IN JEFF'S OWN WORDS

Jeff Oliphant wrote a song about his transformation. He wanted to share it with me and with the readers of *Billion Dollar Smile.*

A NEW ME

I cannot help but stare at the reflection in the window,
As I cruise at an altitude of 30,000 feet.
The clouds make it seem almost dreamlike,
And all that I have left is the memory of the cleft.
This was the opening of my soul,
But now that small opening has been closed
To make my image shine like brand-new.

So when I look, I look again, and I look a third time
Then I smile, and say thank you
To all the males and females
Who made a happy ending for this tale.
And though the past can't be erased
With every look at my face.
I know dreams do come true.

Okay, so you kind of expect your family to love you. But when the girls do too, forget about it! Jeff wasn't dating anyone before his smile makeover, and now he reports that he's getting a lot more attention. Before, he had to win girls over relying solely on his personality. Now, they approach him. He's grateful at least that he was forced to develop his winning personality. It's a great backup plan!

When he's not chasing women or being chased by them, Jeff is an aspiring rap artist who also plays the guitar and keyboard. And his new smile and improved speech have given him a new perspective on his life and his art. Jeff says, "Now I'm just me, 100 percent, all the time. Before, I had to try *more,* if that makes sense, or else people would feel awkward around me."

a butterfly emerges
from her cocoon:
the Kiné Korder story

Kiné Korder is an amazing young woman who, because of her looks, led an amazingly difficult life. Kiné was born with excessive tissue on her lips, making her upper and lower lips unusually large. Kiné was also born with an excessive amount of personality, drive, and curiosity about life. And that's what got her through what anyone would have found to be a tough childhood.

BEFORE THE MAKEOVER

You probably can't imagine how mercilessly Kiné was teased about her lips. Although she says she was happy on the inside, she never smiled because she didn't want to draw more attention to the negative attention she was already getting. Can you imagine always censoring yourself every minute of the day? Kiné was living in her own little prison.

Kiné says growing up she built a shield around herself. She convinced herself the teasing and the curious looks didn't bother her. She said that she put herself under a lot of pressure to maintain that level of denial.

But she was never one to complain—Kiné didn't talk about her problems to anyone. That's because Kiné isn't the sort of person who talks about problems. Kiné talks about solutions and since she didn't have a solution to her smile, she didn't talk about it at all.

But a solution was possible. When Kiné came to me and I told her we could reduce the size of her lower and upper lips, she immediately felt better. She said the fact that a professional wasn't freaked out made her feel like maybe she wasn't so hopeless after all. But I have to say, in over twenty years of practicing dentistry, I had never seen redundant tissue like that before. When the producers of *Extreme Makeover* asked my opinion about whether Kiné would make a good candidate, I pushed for her, knowing it would be a real challenge.

HOW WE FIXED KINÉ'S SMILE

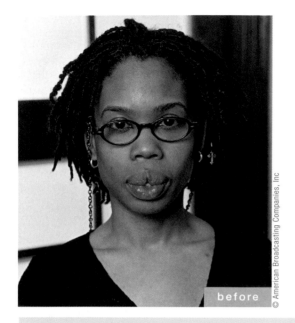
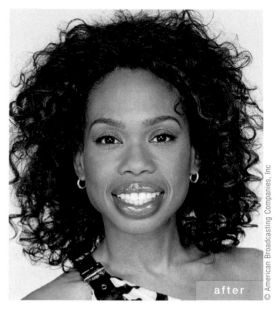

before

after

Kiné Korder's beautiful new smile was achieved through lip surgery, contouring, and ZOOM! whitening.

To give Kiné that Billion Dollar Smile, Dr. Garth Fisher, who was the first plastic surgeon on *Extreme Makeover*, and I did a lip reduction. When that healed, I straightened, whitened, and reshaped her teeth.

Kiné says her smile makeover helped make her inner beauty match her new outer beauty. Before her surgery, she was too guarded: She needed to be in absolute control and shared only a small part of herself with others. By revealing only select parts of herself, she kept the illusion that she could control how others treated her. Only after her smile transformation did she realize what a disservice she had been doing to herself.

Kiné knew that a carefree spirit was in her all along, but she was so busy protecting herself, she didn't let her true self shine. She says her makeover set her free. With her transformation, she discovered happiness is unlimited.

Kiné's attitude toward life has changed. She says, "I used to have to think of profound things to say to distract people from looking at my lips. I used to constantly remind myself, 'Don't be known as the girl with the lips—be known as the smart girl.' Now, I'm just myself."

She learned that some people weren't even aware they were treating her differently because of her appearance. And after she got her new smile, Kiné had an epiphany: Maybe it hadn't *always* been about her lips or about her at all.

One day, after her makeover, Kiné was driving with the windows down and heard a group of people in the car next to her laughing. In the past she would have assumed they were laughing at her lips. It took a moment to realize that she now had a beautiful smile, lips included, so they could not be laughing at her at all. After a few minutes it hit her that things had probably never been as bad as she had thought.

Kiné now finds herself smiling all the time and she's observed that it's infectious. She feels like she lights up a room with her new smile. People are always telling her how lovely her smile is, and her new, brighter spirit is not going unnoticed either.

Today, Kiné shares her bright spirit with others as a life coach and an inspirational speaker (her Web site is www.realimagegroup.com). She is also an actress and a spoken word poet.

Kiné has a very healthy perspective on accepting one's appearance. She says, "Keep the best of you and fix the rest of you." Kiné felt she needed to change her lips to feel whole. For someone else, maximizing his or her best might mean a simple tooth whitening. Everyone sees himself or herself differently.

We all want to be respected, befriended, and loved. But what Kiné has learned is that you have to respect, befriend, and love *yourself* first before expecting that from others. And if you need to change your image of yourself to do that, then go for it!

Another beautiful thing about Kiné's story is that unlike most of the patients on *Extreme Makeover,* she did not require thousands of dollars worth of treatment. All of her dental work and lip surgery probably would have cost less than two thousand dollars. When I asked her why she had not done anything about her lips earlier, she stated that she did not realize anything could be done. Now, not only Kiné but also the millions who watched her know how easily a problem like hers can be fixed.

a killer smile:
the Ray Krone story

I had the honor of helping transform one's man's tragic tale into a story of strength and personal victory. I'm talking about Ray Krone, one of the most inspirational, solid, and sane human beings I've ever been fortunate enough to meet. Ray's Extreme Makeover is, in a way, a makeover for all of us who believe in second chances.

Here was a man who, for years, sat on death row for a murder he did not commit, who refused to be defeated by a system that betrayed him. Ray lost ten years of his life in prison but was exonerated when a DNA test proved his innocence. The only thing he was guilty of was *looking* like a killer.

BEFORE THE MAKEOVER

Ray was called the Snaggletooth Killer because of his scraggly, jagged teeth, which were the result of extensive damage to his mouth in a serious car accident as a teenager. He learned to live with his broken smile. That snaggletooth smile, however, got him more than just jeers and stares—it got him a death sentence.

Ray was wrongly accused of stabbing a female bartender to death. A so-called expert testified that the bite marks on the victim's body matched Ray's teeth, and that the bite mark pattern was as accurate as a fingerprint in identifying him as the only possible suspect. Although Ray had an alibi and there was not a single trace of any other evidence against him, the courts convicted him. Only problem was, they had the wrong man.

Ray says his old smile probably bothered others more than it bothered him. But, in a strange way, it made him a stronger person. He says that when you feel self-conscious about something on the outside, it makes you all that much stronger on the inside. Ray's parents raised him to be a good person and he never doubted who he was, even though people saw him differently.

Being judged for having an unattractive smile is one thing, but being judged as a cold-blooded killer is another. It rocked Ray to the core to be considered a predator, and although he never got used to being unjustly accused, he eventually became somewhat numb to the pain. Somehow, he says, "you learn to swim upstream."

Ray's family believed in him and that made all the difference. Ray was fortunate to make friends in prison too. He was always the kind of guy who helped people out no matter what. Being incarcerated, of course, Ray was forced to ask for legal help. But it wasn't long before he was helping himself, studying the law to help further his case. He became a legal rep for other prisoners, many of whom could not read or write past a grade school level. Eventually DNA evidence cleared Ray, and another man, who later confessed, was convicted of the crime.

When I first saw Ray's teeth (Ray didn't smile much before his makeover, so I can't say that I saw his smile), I understood where that awful snaggletooth moniker came from. Ray's teeth were crooked and painfully out of place. I told him flat out, "Ray, you're a mess. It looks like a bullet went through your mouth." For me, it wasn't just about creating a great smile for Ray—it was about liberating him. But I had a lot of work to do.

HOW WE FIXED RAY'S SMILE

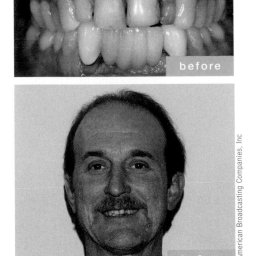

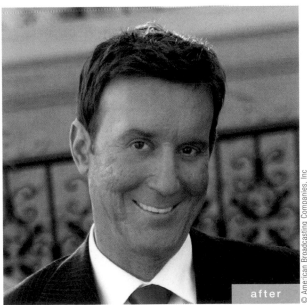

Ray Krone's smile makeover included ZOOM! whitening, implants, crowns, permanent bridges, and veneers.

Ray's mouth was a challenge. I had to extract several of his upper and lower front teeth. We replaced these with implants. Because we were placing crowns, veneers, and permanent bridges on only Ray's front teeth, I used ZOOM! in-office whitening on his back teeth first. This way I could match his new teeth to a lighter shade and have all the teeth match in color.

Compared to the other *Extreme Makeover* participants, Ray took his new smile in stride. He wasn't exactly jumping up and down with joy. At first I was surprised that there were no tears, not even the classic "Oh, my God!" And when Ray's smile reveal was filmed, a producer even said to me, "Man, I thought we'd get a bigger reaction from Ray." However, after putting myself in Ray's place, I responded, "He just spent the last ten years on death row. You think he's going to cry over his teeth?" But after the cameraman and crew had left, as I was walking out of the room, Ray reached out and put his hand on my shoulder. Looking me in the eye, he said, "Doc, you'll never know how much this means to me." It's moments like that one that make my work pay off in spades.

There's a reason for Ray's subdued reaction. To survive the harsh prison environment, he had to learn to keep his feelings suppressed. Ray says his makeover was one of the most special moments in his life, but he didn't want to put on an emotional act for the cameras. He says he wouldn't know how to do that even if he tried.

But when Ray got home and was finally alone, the floodgates opened. His makeover stirred something deep inside him. It started a tremor within him, a tremor that became an earthquake, and that's when the tears came. In a lot of ways, Ray's new life began right then and there, after his makeover, not after his release from prison.

For the first time since his arrest, he began to feel that the world was aligning back on its axis. I feel fortunate to have been able, in some sense, to give Ray his freedom. Without a new smile, every time Ray looked at himself, his teeth would have reminded him of an awful chapter in his life.

So what does Ray think of second chances? Ray says there's a certain feeling of liberation in not searching for what was lost. He lost ten years of his life in prison but doesn't want to look back. He says what happened to him was someone else's fault. What happens now is his own responsibility.

Having a killer smile, pun intended, will only help Ray. He is putting his new smile to good use as an inspirational speaker and anti-death-penalty advocate. Ray says he's still trying to figure out who Ray Krone is while looking forward.

It is disturbing to realize that what happened to Ray Krone could happen to any of us. Ray played Little League, got good grades, and never even spent time in detention. He served in the Air Force and held down a good job as a postal worker.

Before I met Ray, I saw the death penalty issue in black and white. It wasn't until Diane Sawyer unexpectedly confronted me on *Good Morning America* about my uncle who was stabbed to death that I realized that Ray and I had something in common. I used to believe in the Old Testament verse: "An eye for an eye and a tooth for a tooth." I believed if you killed someone, then you deserved to die. End of story. But after meeting Ray Krone and hearing his close-call tale, I've reconsidered my position. Mistakes are made and innocent lives are lost. Ray Krone speaks to that truth. Unfortunately, the death penalty doesn't allow for mistakes. Ray Krone is living, breathing, and smiling proof that we might need to rethink how our legal system works.

smile doubles: the Caroline Johnson and Catherine Bunnell story

When they were kids no one could tell them apart, but as they matured into women, identical twins Caroline and Catherine (called Cat) didn't look identical anymore.

Caroline and Cat came on *Extreme Makeover* because they wanted to look more like each other again. In junior high they both had braces, but after their parents' divorce there was no money for "luxuries" such as orthodontics. Cat had worn her braces longer than her sister, so her teeth were better off. But Caroline had to have her braces removed after only six months. As a result, Caroline's teeth began a downward spiral. Because they were so crooked, it was difficult to keep them clean and they started to decay all over. In addition, she had a very gummy smile. And if crooked teeth were not bad enough, Caroline broke her nose, so that was crooked too.

Caroline says she felt like the ugly duckling next to Cat. Cat says it wasn't any easier for her. She said she always felt uncomfortable and sorry for her sister.

HOW WE FIXED THE TWINS' SMILES

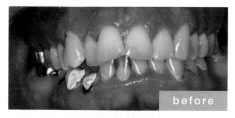

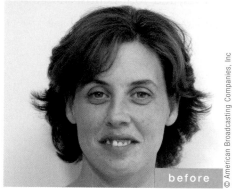

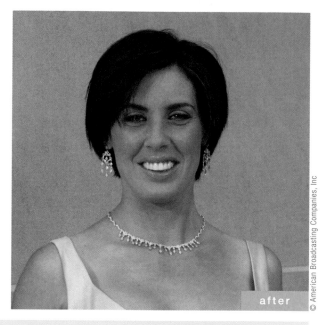

To improve her smile, Caroline Johnson needed lip repositioning, ZOOM! whitening, crowns or veneers on almost every tooth, and gum recontouring.

We gave Caroline extensive dental work including ZOOM! in-office whitening, twenty-four porcelain veneers and crowns, lip repositioning surgery, gum recontouring, and two root canals. And, of course, the plastic surgeon repaired her broken nose. Cat also needed some work, including eight upper porcelain veneers, ZOOM! in-office whitening, gum recontouring, and orthodontics to straighten the lower teeth.

When people ask Caroline what I did for her, she says, "What *didn't* he do for me?" In fact, if I had worked on Caroline in dental school, I could have fulfilled all of my requirements on her alone! In addition to working on her teeth, to get rid of her gummy smile we did a lip repositioning procedure—lowering her upper lip—and a crown lengthening procedure in which we removed or surgically contoured her excess gum tissue, essentially raising her gum line. This combination of veneers and gum recontouring gave her normal size teeth without a gummy smile. Even if your teeth are already pretty and positioned correctly, if you see gums, it's not a pretty package.

Of every two hundred minutes of tape for *Extreme Makeover*, only one minute ends up on television. For Caroline it was about a seven-and-a-half-hour procedure for her dental treatment. Afterwards she said, "Oh, they're nice." I thought, "Nice? That's all you have to say?" She looked gorgeous but was drained, and the next day she really appreciated her new smile.

Caroline says working with my team was a completely different experience from working with the dentists from her past, who had always blamed her for her teeth problems. I make it a point to treat all my patients like celebrities, and your dentist should too.

Now the twins look identical again. Cat says, "When I see Caroline smile, I see myself smile." Isn't that sweet?

HOW TO AFFORD DENTAL WORK

If you don't have a lot of money and didn't have the bad "teeth genes" and good luck necessary to be selected for *Extreme Makeover,* there are ways to get dental work for free or at least at reduced rates. Free clinics and dental schools offer assistance to those with limited means. Victims of domestic violence can contact the Give Back a Smile program at www.aacd.com for free dental care. It may not be for extreme cosmetic work, but these resources may be able to help you through a dental crisis or give you more affordable options.

Ask a dentist's office for suggestions or go online and check with dental schools and clinics in your area for more information.

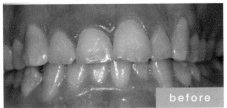

before

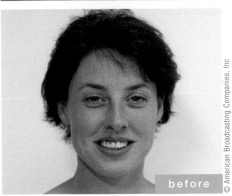

before

© American Broadcasting Companies, Inc

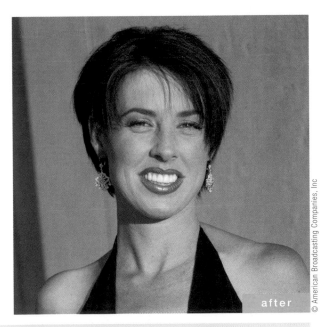

after

© American Broadcasting Companies, Inc

Caroline's twin sister, Catherine (Cat) Bunnell, received ZOOM! whitening, upper porcelain veneers, gum recontouring, and orthodontic treatment.

Caroline's husband, Mark Johnson, says he feels like I was "the other man" but he's okay with that. With three young children, money was tight so Caroline had done without dental treatment and had sacrificed her looks for her family. She says her new smile improved her self-confidence and even strengthened her marriage by reducing the stress of wondering where the money would come from for her teeth. Mark even went as far as to say it was a miracle.

Caroline says she worries that smiling too hard might ruin all the work I did. I say, go for it! Smile away, Caroline.

motor mouth mike: the Michael Cunningham story

Michael Cunningham was a real car nut with one messed up "grille" of a smile. As an auto body mechanic in Vegas, Mike gives cars a makeover for a living and was just as eager to have one himself. And, boy, did he get one.

BEFORE THE MAKEOVER

Mike actually went through life trying *not* to smile. And you really couldn't blame him. His teeth were discolored and crooked. He says they looked like those phony teeth you buy for Halloween costumes. But his smile problems didn't end there. Mike also had a very gummy smile with enough gum tissue for three mouths.

Mike's smile, or lack of a smile, had a huge impact on his personal life. His self-esteem was in the pits. At the age of twenty-one, he had had only one girlfriend and that had lasted only a few days.

HOW WE FIXED MIKE'S SMILE

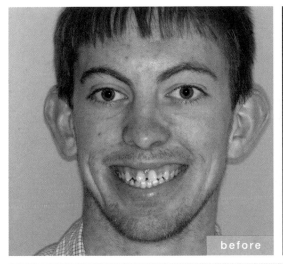
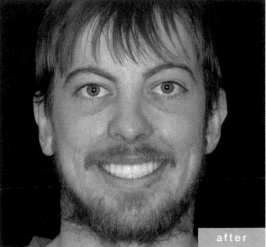

before

after

Mike Cunningham's Extreme Makeover included lip repositioning, crown lengthening, and upper and lower porcelain veneers.

Mike wasn't a demanding patient. He told me he only wanted to look average. Imagine only wanting to look average! The other Extreme Team doctors and I weren't going to settle for that. So we got to work.

I had the periodontist do crown lengthening and lip repositioning to show less of Mike's gums. I then designed for Mike a straight, masculine smile out of porcelain veneers. It was as if I were working in the chop shop and Mike was the car. In all, Mike had lip and gum repositioning plus ZOOM! in-office whitening and sixteen porcelain veneers. He also bulked up his muscles and had acne laser treatment, a nose job, and his ears pinned back.

Mike says he's in love with his new smile. And now he's in love! Mike says, "I like the new me. My confidence has skyrocketed. Now, nothing can hold me back." Mike now feels free to be himself and no longer worries about people judging him based on his appearance. People can finally see him for who he really is. Before, Mike got the sense people didn't really get the chance to know him, and he suspects it had a lot to do with the fact that he never smiled.

Now he comes across as the friendly guy he really is. At the body shop they even call him "Smiley."

the smile stud:
the Eric Rice story

Some say Eric Rice is a stud: an L.A. firefighter by day and hockey player by night. But his smile reduced him to a mere mortal. Eric had lost teeth after being hit in the mouth several times with a hockey stick. His upper lip was also scarred and nonsymmetrical. Eric's lip hung down over the right side of his teeth; this meant he had to smile harder so the lip would "stand up." It looked like he had paralysis on one side of his face.

BEFORE THE MAKEOVER

Eric had lots of work done on his mouth over the years, but none of the new teeth matched his other teeth. So he had a lot of differently shaped and colored teeth.

Eric also wore what we called a flipper, a retainer-like appliance that can replace missing teeth, which he took out at night. This became an occupational hazard for him as a firefighter—a couple of times he showed up at emergencies in the middle of the night with no teeth and scared the heck out of people.

Once he was half an hour late for a date because he left the house without his teeth and had to drive back home to get them—good move.

But even with a messed-up smile, Eric was still a great-looking guy, and not someone you'd expect to see on *Extreme Makeover*. He really only needed a smile makeover. When he walked into my office, my lab technician, Juliet, said, "Dr. Dorfman, is this guy an *Extreme Makeover* patient? I can't believe it. He's so good-looking, what could they possibly be doing to him?"

I couldn't resist. I told her with a straight face that Eric was going to be the first *Extreme Makeover* patient to have a male organ enhancement. Being the joker that he is, Eric chimed in and made the story believable. And Juliet obviously couldn't resist sharing this with every other woman in my office and the entire da Vinci dental lab. Each time Eric came back to my office the girls looked at him oddly. Juliet wanted to know how we would do the reveal to his family and friends on *Extreme Makeover*. I made up a funny scenario and told her she just had to watch the show. Well, she tuned in, along with all her friends and family, and the next morning she wanted to smack me. I deserved it!

HOW WE FIXED ERIC'S SMILE

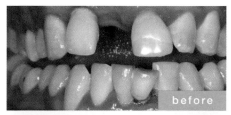
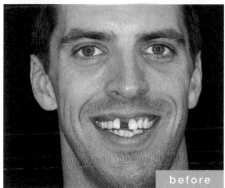
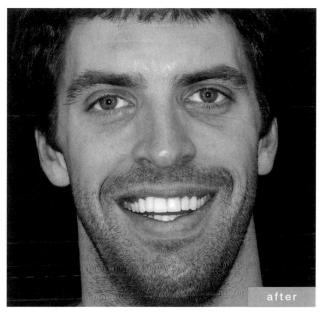

For his handsome new smile, Eric Rice needed scar revision of his lip, lip repositioning, ZOOM! whitening, implants, and crowns or veneers on all his front teeth.

All kidding aside, Eric needed extensive dental work including dental implants, removing the scar tissue from his lip to make it symmetrical, porcelain veneers, lip repositioning surgery, and ZOOM! in-office whitening. Eric was lucky that we were able to help him because when your teeth get extracted or knocked out, the bone holding those teeth in starts to diminish—it simply melts away. And because the bone often shrinks, you should try to get implants right away after losing teeth. It's a use-it-or-lose-it kind of thing. I've seen patients who've actually fractured their jaws while eating because the bone is so thin in the lower jaw after tooth loss that it breaks easily.

Through implants and lip surgery we made Eric's smile symmetrical again. When he saw his new smile, he was stunned. He couldn't even believe it was him. He was used to seeing himself with discolored and missing teeth.

Eric's new smile looks like a billion bucks. He promised me he will always wear a mouth guard on the ice! Eric says most of the hockey players he knows don't even wear mouth guards because they think it's a hassle, and they think they're too cool for masks as well. He gets called a wimp for wearing a mouth guard, but most of the guys giving him grief are missing teeth themselves.

I said to him when it was all done, "You'd better wear that mouth guard I made for you when you play, because if you don't I'm not sure I'll make you a second set!"

the sixty-thousand dollar smile: the Kim Rodriguez story

Most of us take smiling for granted. But when I first met Kim Rodriguez, she swore to me she could not smile.

Kim said, "Honestly, Dr. Dorfman, I don't how to smile. I honestly don't." When she tried, it looked like she was in pain. She was. Not physical pain, but an even more painful emotional torment.

BEFORE THE MAKEOVER

Kim wanted to correct a terrible overbite and desperately needed to replace missing and broken teeth. She never had braces as a child and it broke her parents' hearts that they couldn't afford to fix their little girl's smile.

Despite her situation, Kim made the proverbial lemonade out of lemons and grew up to be a confident, hard-working adult. But she could never quite get over her teeth. Kim said she never, ever smiled unless she kept her mouth closed. If she burst into laughter, she'd cover her teeth with her hand. She lived every minute bound by this constant reminder that her smile was inadequate. She said that as a result she felt inadequate too.

Kim wanted a second chance. She was terrified of meeting new people, afraid they would judge her or dismiss her because of her appearance. She would literally "practice" how to hide her smile in front of the mirror. It was that important to her to keep her teeth her secret.

HOW WE FIXED KIM'S SMILE

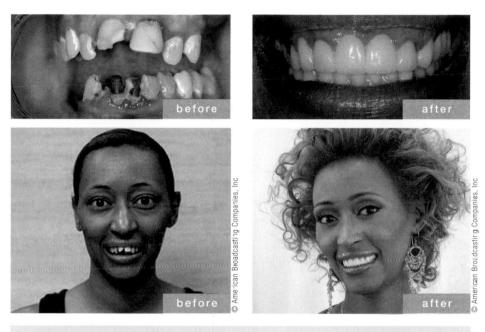

Kim Rodriguez's Extreme Makeover included lip repositioning, crown lengthening, upper and lower permanent bridges, removable partial dentures, and crowns or veneers on every tooth.

Kim was selected from thousands of hopefuls for *Extreme Makeover,* and when she first sat down in my chair, I asked her to open her mouth so I could see what we were dealing with. I literally jumped back when I saw her teeth. The teeth that hadn't fallen out jutted out at a forty-degree angle. They were crumbling and ready to fall out.

I extracted six front teeth (two uppers and four lowers) and gave Kim lip repositioning, gum repositioning (crown lengthening), upper and lower permanent bridges, removable partial dentures, a few root canals, porcelain veneers, and crowns. Whew! What a job, about sixty thousand dollars worth of dentistry, but worth every teardrop that Kim cried when she saw them. Between hugging me and looking in the mirror, she kept repeating over and over how beautiful they were.

At her reveal, her family and friends were just as awestruck. Everyone was staring at her brilliant new smile. And Kim loved every second. She said, "What Dr. Dorfman did for me was give me back my life. Thank you just isn't enough. I always knew I was beautiful inside and now I feel complete."

When the episode aired, ABC put Kim's face up on the huge screen in New York's Times Square, where she lit the whole square up. In fact, after lighting up Times Square, Kim said she felt like her smile could light up the world.

the gobble sisters: the Frannie Dodrill, Jennie Martinson, and Katye Lent story

Frannie Dodrill, Jennie Martinson, and Katye Lent called themselves the Gobble sisters, a derogatory self-reference to what they called their turkey necks, excess skin on their necks. They should call themselves the "I want to gobble you up sisters." These three women were the funniest, sweetest, most wonderful sisters I've ever had the pleasure of treating. To them, I'm Billy. Thanks, Mom. (That's what my mother calls me, and after the sisters met her, they picked up on it.)

The three came to L.A. for their Extreme Makeovers as part of a package deal. Their kids made them do it. All three looked a lot older than their ages, and their children decided it was time their mothers did something for themselves, for once.

When all was said and done, I did forty-eight porcelain veneers on the three sisters. You do the math! Frannie says, "We literally have Billion Dollar Smiles!"

FRANNIE'S STORY

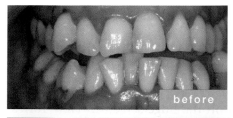

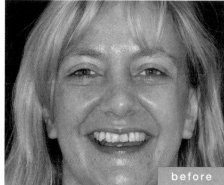

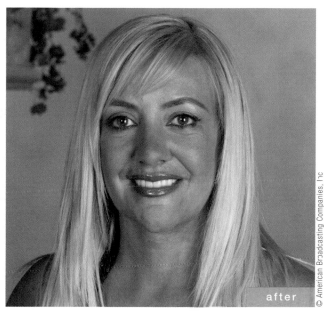

Frannie Dodrill's Billion Dollar smile included extensive gum surgery, ZOOM! whitening, and upper and lower porcelain veneers.

Let's start with Frannie and her "fang" —a canine tooth that stuck out. She hated it and wanted it gone. Actually, it didn't have to "go" anywhere. To minimize how far it stuck out, I filed it down and placed a porcelain veneer on it. It was like instant orthodontics.

But that was only the beginning. I designed Frannie's Billion Dollar Smile using fifteen other porcelain veneers. I also performed a root canal and major gum surgery. It seemed like I did an Extreme Makeover just on her gums!

During it all, Frannie's dental drama was intensified by another one of her sisters, one who was not featured on the show. Frannie kept begging me to just take all her teeth out and give her dentures because her older sister, who had suffered periodontal disease, had been advising her to get rid of her real teeth. I got a frantic phone call one night from Frannie pleading with me, saying, "Dr. Dorfman, you're a nice guy but just take them out!"

I said, "No way! Give me a chance." (I felt like we were dating!) I insisted we could save her teeth and place veneers over them. Frannie was concerned that even if we did save them now, she could not afford to maintain them. I promised her that if she came back to L.A every three to four months, I would continue to take care of her teeth. Frannie now says she was grateful she listened to me and her new smile is a "miracle." She says, "I was just waiting for my teeth to all fall out someday. To be able to smile and laugh now is huge. I can't even tell you how I feel."

Frannie's new smile and whole new look made her feel younger and more attractive than ever. She reports that she posted her new "Barbie doll" picture of herself on some Internet dating sites and found a great guy.

JENNIE'S STORY

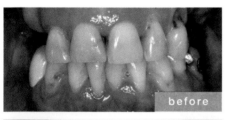
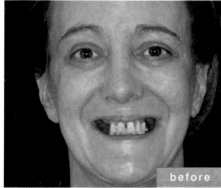
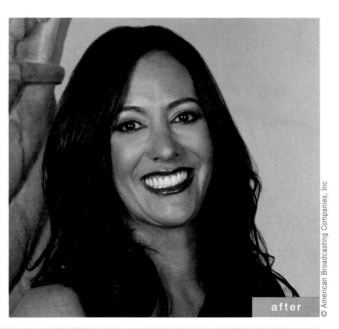

Jennie Martinson's gorgeous new smile was the result of gum surgery, porcelain veneers, and upper and lower removable partial dentures.

Jennie works in a gold mine. Now that she's had a smile makeover, her bright smile is probably the only thing they can see down in the mine! She explained that when the sisters were younger, they weren't taught proper dental hygiene. It was obvious Jennie was also the victim of some pretty bad dental care, leaving her with a smile that made her look twenty years older than she was. In fact, Jennie said that's how long it was since she'd smiled in public. She felt like it was hopeless, and that her smile made her look ugly. She had tried to get her teeth capped, but her dentists said it wasn't worth it, so she was basically just waiting for them to fall out so she could get dentures.

Jennie had the worst teeth of the sisters. Every time her dentist told her it was either a root canal or an extraction, she got a tooth pulled because it was cheaper. As a mother raising three children, she couldn't justify paying thousands more in dental bills when she had sneakers to buy for her kids.

When she came to my office with her sisters for their Extreme Makeover, Jennie said, "You can help my sisters but you probably can't help me." But *can't* is a word I don't understand.

Jennie said she thought makeovers were superficial. The only thing she really wanted done was her teeth. I gave her fifteen porcelain veneers, upper and lower removable partial dentures, a root canal, and gum surgery. As you can see from Jennie's "after" photographs, her brand-new smile completely changed her appearance. She looks like she could be the daughter of the person in her "before" photo.

Jennie says now she smiles all the time. She says, "When you really smile, I mean really smile, you get a great feeling in your heart. I feel so much better all the time now."

Jennie is looking forward to a new life with her new smile, but jokes that she never wants anyone to forget the "old Jennie." She keeps an old photograph of herself on her refrigerator door to remind everyone that she's still one tough lady. "Don't mess with me," she jokes, "because this is how I look on the inside!"

KATYE'S STORY

The third sister, Katye, was affectionately called Gumby by her family. When she smiled, it was all gums. I gave Katye seventeen porcelain veneers, a root canal, and lip repositioning. I tacked her upper lip down so that when she smiles, less gum is revealed. She's not called Gumby anymore!

Katye says now strangers stop her in the supermarket and tell her she has the most beautiful smile. Receiving compliments is something she has to get used to. She says, "I've never experienced it before. It's quite an adjustment and I like it."

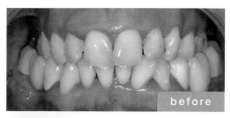

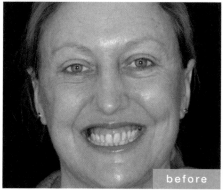

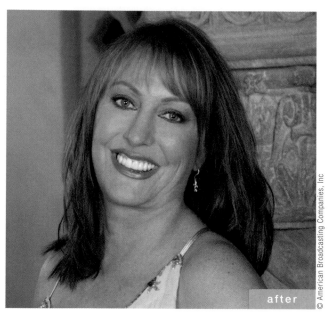

Katye Lent's smile makeover included porcelain veneers and lip repositioning.

Katye is now the self-described "dating queen" of the three sisters. She says she didn't date for three whole years before her smile makeover, and now she's having so much fun she doesn't want to settle down. Now this forty-something mom is turning down guys in their twenties.

CONQUERING FEAR

But these new smiles didn't come easy—for me or for the three sisters! One thing all three women had to conquer was their fear of dentists.

Jennie says she was scared to death. She wanted new teeth but was petrified. The biggest challenge was getting her comfortable and getting her to believe that after it was all done she was going to walk out with a beautiful smile.

It wasn't just a fear of pain, but bad bedside manner from former dentists that made Jennie's discomfort worse. She said dentists had blamed her for her bad teeth and made her feel like it was her fault she was born with a less-than-perfect smile.

But the ladies got over their fears and put their trust in me. I held their hands and explained every procedure every step of the way. When it was all over, the sisters celebrated their new smiles and bodies by going on a "love cruise"—unfortunately, I was not invited on the trip. The only details of the cruise they would share with me were that they met a bunch of sexy firefighters. The sisters said they had an amazing time creating a lot of heat!

you get what you pay for: the Missy Madrid story

In the beginning Missy Madrid (great name!) might have acted like a stalker, but she turned out to be a determined patient and later a great friend. Missy is a fantastic, warm, caring woman from Midland, Texas, who reached out to me via e-mail about her dental nightmare. She was a big fan of *Extreme Makeover* who watched me transform dozens of smiles and became motivated to improve her own smile.

THE BOTCHED MAKEOVER

Missy is a cautionary tale for cheap cosmetic surgery. For the price I charge for one veneer, she had her whole smile made over by an inexperienced dentist in another country. Missy's botched smile makeover nearly incapacitated her with pain and depression. After her ordeal, Missy wrote me asking for help. After reading several of her e-mails, I finally called her and tried to set her up with a dentist in her area. But she wanted only me—how could I say no?

Missy never had great teeth to begin with. She had a nice smile but her teeth were discolored from fluorosis caused by too much fluoride intake as a child. Fluoride is beneficial in moderation, but like lots of things in life, too much of a good thing is not good. In Missy's case it caused white and brown spots and created pits on her teeth, making irregular surfaces. But that didn't keep Missy from smiling or enjoying life.

Missy was married to her college sweetheart, Ronn, and had two wonderful boys. Eventually, she felt she needed a smile makeover. She wanted her husband and sons to be proud of her.

But Missy and her husband didn't have a lot of money. They were hard-working people with bills to pay and kids "fixing" (as she says) to go off to college, so money was tight.

So Missy decided to go across the border from her home in Texas to a clinic in Mexico. The problems began as soon as she sat down in the chair. Her dentist did not speak English, so communication was limited to pointing and gesturing. Not a good start when collaborating on a smile makeover.

From the moment they drilled her teeth "down to little nubs" she knew she was in trouble. Missy had asked for conservative veneers but because of the communication problem, she got crowns—and not good ones. You could see the metal up around her gum line. Her "after" in her first smile makeover was actually worse than her "before."

On top of that, the bite didn't match so she couldn't close her mouth properly. Missy says she couldn't sleep at night because of the pain. She was afraid to eat in public, and even to eat in front of her family. She got very depressed and cried all the time.

She was in constant pain and discomfort. The caps never fit properly and they looked unnatural. They were a dull gray, not a natural color for teeth. They were too bulky and they leaked around her teeth. Her gums were swollen and bleeding because the caps didn't fit properly.

But things got worse. The caps began falling off. The ones that remained caused a lot of pain because liquid leaked inside the caps and irritated the roots. Exposed dentin can be very sensitive—it's worse than walking outside in bitter cold without a coat.

Missy sent me an e-mail asking me to help her. Because of *Extreme Makeover* and because I lecture around the world, I get hundreds of these letters, but what stood out for me was the fact that she kept saying how she used to have such a happy life, with a loving soulmate for a husband and two teenage boys. It wasn't the usual "Debbie Downer" kind of letter.

Her new teeth were the roadblock in her otherwise happy life. She said they made her miserable. In addition to pain, Missy felt guilt because she had brought it all on herself and her family when her old teeth were not that bad to begin with.

THE REAL MAKEOVER

Missy was shocked when I called her at home. She cried her eyes out and barely got a word in. I tried to calm her down and told her everything was going to be all right,

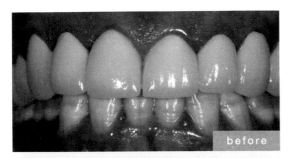
before

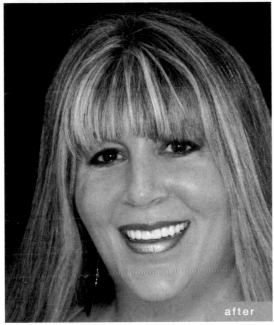
after

Missy Madrid's new makeover consisted of all-porcelain crowns on the upper arch and porcelain veneers on the lower arch to match the uppers.

that I'd help her find a dentist in Texas to help her.

But she said, no, she wanted only me to do it, especially after dentists had told her that fixing her smile was going to be expensive and painful, "like sticking a jackhammer to your face." So she insisted on coming to my office in the Beverly Hills area. Missy said she'd sell her truck to finance her new smile if necessary.

And I told her not to be ridiculous, that we'd figure out a way to make this affordable for her. I gave Missy twelve upper porcelain crowns and twelve lower veneers. My makeover, which was basically a makeover of her botched makeover, took eight hours the first day and another eight hours the second day. It did the trick.

When it was over, Missy said she looked like she had a movie star's mouth. When she saw her new smile, Missy and her husband sat in the car and cried. They were so relieved. She got her life back and Ronn got his wife back.

Missy says she's grateful to God and she believes he answered her prayers. She tells me she's started to feel like herself again.

A beautiful smile is not just about vanity. It is an indication of one's health and well-being. Your smile is an essential trait in communication and is often a manifestation of socioeconomic status. Time and time again patients from all walks of life state that when their broken smiles are restored they feel a sense of completion. For many it is the critical missing piece of the puzzle that allows them to feel whole. Having a beautiful smile is liberating, and we all know that when you smile the whole world smiles with you.

afterword

Charity work has always been a big part of my life. I am eternally grateful for all that I have and I feel it's important to give back. With my business partner Robert Hayman, CEO of Discus Dental; our company, Discus Dental; and a network of dentists in the Crown Council, directed by Greg Anderson from Salt Lake City, I have been working since the late 1990s with the Smiles for Life Foundation (www.smilesforlife.org), which donates funds to many children's charities. You may have seen or heard me or my friend Garth Brooks, the legendary country singer, doing public service announcements talking about ways to brighten a child's smile and help that child "smile for life." Calling the organization's number, 877-FOR SMILES, connects you with the closest participating dentist in your area who is a member of the Crown Council organization. For a four-month period every year, you can get your teeth whitened at a reduced rate by a Crown Council participating dentist—and your entire payment goes straight to Smiles for Life. This program was initiated by Crown Council member Dr. Jeff Gray.

When Smiles for Life initially contacted Discus Dental, we were asked to sell our products to the foundation at cost. However, we decided to provide our whitening products—Nite White, Day White, and ZOOM!—for free so that more money could go to the kids. In our second year, Discus Dental joined with Garth Brooks's Teammates for Kids Foundation and let Garth's organization distribute the majority of the money.

In the last six years, we raised more than $20 million for cancer research, inner-city schools, dental care, research, and treatment for kids with catastrophic diseases.

I don't need to tell you that children in need extend beyond our backyard. That's why I also participate in CHOICE, the Center for Humanitarian Outreach and Inter-Cultural Exchange (www.choicehumanitarian.org). CHOICE dentists, led by Dr. Roy Hammond, travel to different parts of the world to provide dental care for needy children.

In Mexico we went to three different locations and treated nearly five hundred kids in less than a week. We went to villages without electricity, so in addition to our own instruments, equipment, and dental supplies, we had to supply our own generators.

When we visited an orphanage for blind and medically compromised children, I brought my eldest daughter, Anna, who was nine at the time. I was so proud of her; she helped put the children's fears to rest by playing with them, painting their faces, holding their hands, and blowing the rubber gloves up into balloons. While she distracted them, we filled cavities, pulled teeth, and even bonded teeth. The way I see it, for every cavity we filled, we saved that tooth. Without dental care the teeth would have continued to decay until they fell out. We also taught the children to brush and floss because prevention is key.

My main goal was to help the children, but my ulterior motive was to help my child appreciate what we have and how important it is to make a difference in the world and make it a better place. I wanted my daughter to see that I just don't say it, I do it.

The most exciting project we are working on is for The National Children's Dental Foundation (TNCDF). For years we have been supporting The Children's Dental Center in Los Angeles, which offers dental care to children of the working poor. Dental disease is the number-one childhood ailment, and many of these children have nowhere else to go for dental care. Because of the success we have had with this center, we are using it as a prototype to help build five hundred centers all over the USA in the next five years. We project that we will be able to treat more than 20 million children in this five-year period.

I also offer assistance to women from the Los Angeles Battered Women's Shelter. Most of the women I worked on had lost their teeth to domestic violence and could not afford to replace them. To protect their privacy and dignity, no one except my office manager and I know their situations, and they are treated like regular, paying patients.

The women go through a twelve-step program before they leave the shelter. One of the women (who graciously permitted me to mention her here) had a really difficult time finding a job, so I hired her as an entry-level receptionist at Discus Dental. She was sweet and friendly, and she's since moved on to a higher-level job in another company. While I was proud of her "moving on up," it was hard to let her go. Every morning when I walked into work she greeted me with the sweetest, "God bless you, Dr. Dorfman." I called her Sunshine because she was so radiant.

I'm not suggesting a new smile solved these women's problems, but it was one missing link that helped them go out into the world again. A smile helped make them feel whole.

Anyone can start over—and a new smile can give you the chance to reinvent yourself, to begin anew. No matter where you are or where you want to be in your life, I believe a beautiful smile can make a big difference.

glossary

Abrasion: Erosion of tooth structure

ADA: American Dental Association

AACD: American Academy of Cosmetic Dentists

Bonding: Using tooth-colored resin material (composite) to fill in or reshape teeth; see *composite*

Bridge: An artificial fixed or removable appliance to replace missing natural teeth

Bruxism: Grinding of teeth, usually worse at night

Calculus: Hard calcium matter, also called *tartar*, which is deposited on teeth

Cap: An artificial tooth covering that covers all the way around the entire tooth; also called *crown*

Cavity: A hole in enamel, and in some cases dentin, caused by decay

Composite: The tooth-colored material used to fill cavities or to bond to teeth; see *bonding*

Contouring: Shaping teeth for a more appealing smile

Crown: An artificial tooth covering that covers all the way around the tooth; also called *cap*

Cuspid: The third tooth on either side of the midline; also called a *canine*

Decay: The deterioration of teeth from the acid produced by bacteria

Dentin: The hard tooth structure directly beneath the enamel

Dentophobia: Fear of dentists and dental procedures

Dentures: Artificial teeth that replace part or all of an entire mouth of teeth

Enamel: The outermost hard layer of teeth

Endodontist: A dentist who specializes in root canals

Erosion: The wearing away of tooth structure because of excessive brushing or chemical causes

Fixed bridge: Artificial teeth that are permanently cemented onto surrounding teeth to replace missing teeth or to splint loose teeth; also called *permanent bridge*

Fluoride: Found in most city water supplies and in toothpaste; a binary compound of fluorine and another element; makes teeth harder and more resistant to cavities

Gingivitis: Redness, swelling, and inflammation of the gums; if untreated, can progress to periodontitis (gum disease)

Halitosis: Chronic bad breath

Halitometer: A sulfide monitor that gauges the gases in breath

Hygienist: A dental professional who specializes in teeth cleaning and maintenance of teeth

Implants: Metal fixtures placed into the bone, which become the base for artificial tooth replacement

Incisors: The four upper and lower front teeth

Laminate: A conservative porcelain or resin covering that mainly covers the front of teeth to change the color, size, or position, or to fill in spaces; also called *veneer*

Malocclusion: An overbite, underbite, or unnatural bite where teeth are not lined up properly

Midline: The midpoint of the face

Orthodontist: A dentist who specializes in orthodontia (braces) or the movement of teeth

Orthognathic surgery: Surgical treatment to correct the malposition of the jawbones

Osseointegration: The biological attachment of a metallic implant to bone with no intervening connective tissue

Periodontist: A dentist who specializes in gums, bone, and the support structure of teeth

Periodontitis: A disease characterized by inflammation of the gums, which leads to irreversible loss of bone structure

Permanent bridge: Artificial teeth that are permanently cemented onto surrounding teeth to replace missing teeth or to splint loose teeth; also called *fixed bridge*

Plaque: Bacteria that stick to the teeth and can cause decay if not removed

Pontic: An artificial tooth attached to a bridge where there is no root or support under it

Pulp: Nerves and tissue in the tooth core

Restoration: The replacement or reinforcement of tooth structure with materials found in fillings, bonding, crowns, bridges, veneers, and so on.

Root canal: A procedure to remove diseased or dead tissue from teeth so the tooth can be restored

Rotations: Teeth that are not in alignment or are "twisted"

Tartar: A hard, destructive substance that forms on teeth as a result of plaque buildup that calcifies; also called *calculus*

Temporaries: Short-term tooth replacements usually worn while a permanent restoration is made

Tetracycline: An antibiotic that can discolor teeth

Veneer: A conservative porcelain or resin covering that mainly covers the front of teeth to change the color, size, or position, or to fill in spaces; also called *laminate*

index

BreathRx (breath control system), xiii, 134–135, 142, 146, 151

Bridges

care of, 81

Maryland bridges, 80

permanent bridges, 3, 79–82, 175, 181–182, 191

procedure for, 80–81

pros and cons of, 81

purpose of, 79

removable bridges, 82–85

BriteSmile, xiii

Brodsky, Marla, xv

Broken smiles, 7

Brooks, Garth, 201

Brushing teeth, 128–131, 133, 137, 146, 151

Bruxism, 15, 53, 140–142

Bulimia, 145, 147

Bunnell, Catherine, 183–185

Burnett, Mark, 160

C

Calcium, 142

Calculus (tartar), 129–130, 133

Candy, 144–145, 146

Canine teeth, 18–37

Caps. *See* Crowns

Carbohydrates, 144

Cavities, 135–136, 138–139, 144–145

Celebrities

as patients, xiii, 157–163

requested smiles of, 39

smile types, 40–51, 54–62

Center for Humanitarian Outreach and Inter-Cultural Exchange (CHOICE), 201–202

Central incisors, 18–37

Cervantes, Miguel de, xiv

Chairside bleaching, 120–121. *See also* ZOOM! Chairside Whitening System

Charity work, 201–203

Chewing gum, 130, 142, 146, 151, 155

Children, oral hygiene routines for, 137–138

Children's Dental Center (Los Angeles), 202

CHOICE (Center for Humanitarian Outreach and Inter-Cultural Exchange), 201–202

Clear braces, 103–104

Cleft lip and palate, 2, 3, 83, 174–175

Clip-on dentures, 89, 92–93

Clooney, George, 46

Cole Fenton, Jennifer, xiv

Composite fillings, 124, 136

Composite veneers, 75–77

Concealed braces, 104–105

Contouring, 67–69

Cosmetic dentistry

advances in, xii, xv

artistic aspect of, 8, 9, 106

bargain dental centers, 146

benefits of, 1

choosing a dentist, 166–168

confidence from, xvi, 4

cost of procedures, xii, xiii, 185, 191

free and reduced-rate work, 185

limiting factors, 17

purpose of, 7

quality of, 198

types of procedures, 65–66

whitening teeth and, 114

Cosmetic surgery, xii, xvi, 8

about the authors

Dr. Bill Dorfman

Dr. Bill Dorfman's patient roster includes some of Hollywood's brightest stars: Alanis Morissette, Brooke Burke, Sean Astin, Ozzy Osbourne and family, Usher, Jessica Simpson, Nick Lachey, Debra Messing, and Hugh Jackman, to name a few.

Affectionately known as Dr. Bill, Dr. Dorfman has brought award-winning innovations to aesthetic dentistry. He has been consulted extensively for numerous television and magazine interviews, and has a featured role on ABC's mega-hit series, *Extreme Makeover,* which won a 2006 People's Choice Award and is seen in over one hundred countries around the world.

Dr. Dorfman is also featured in the Learning Channel's *Ten Years Younger* makeover show and he's seen all over the UK on Channel 5's *Brand New You.* He has appeared on *Oprah, The Tonight Show with Jay Leno, Larry King Live, The Today Show,* MTV's *The Newlyweds, The Osbournes, Good Morning America, Entertainment Tonight, The View, E! Entertainment Television, The Tyra Banks Show, The Janice Dickinson Modeling Agency, Reality Remix, Cold Turkey, The Rosie O'Donnell Show,* and others.

He graduated from UCLA and received his dental degree in 1983 from the University of the Pacific in San Francisco, and completed a two-year residency at a dental hospital in Lausanne, Switzerland. In 1985 Dr. Dorfman established his private practice in aesthetic and general dentistry in the Beverly Hills area.

In 1989, at age thirty, Dr. Dorfman founded Discus Dental, Inc., the world's leading manufacturer and distributor of tooth whitening, oral hygiene, and aesthetic dental products. Here he helped develop award-winning take-home teeth whitening products such as Nite White and Day White. Discus Dental also launched ZOOM!, the number one in-office whitening system in the world, and has acquired BriteSmile, another popular in-office professional whitening system. Dr. Dorfman and Discus Dental are also responsible for BreathRx, the leading line of dentist-supplied breath-freshening products, which is now available online and in retail stores.

Dr. Dorfman is a member of the American Dental Association and the Century City Medical Staff, and is one of only thirty-three Fellows in the American Academy of Cosmetic Dentistry. He is a world-renowned lecturer and author of one of the best-selling books on cosmetic dentistry, *The Smile Guide*. He is also the past editor of the *Journal of the American Academy of Cosmetic Dentistry*.

In addition, Dr. Dorfman was the founder and program coordinator of PAC-live, a continuing education program to teach practicing dentists state-of-the-art cosmetic dental skills on live patients, at the Arthur A. Dugoni School of Dentistry at the University of the Pacific in San Francisco. He has been honored as the "Best Aesthetic Dentist in Los Angeles" in *Los Angeles Magazine*, and was awarded five lifetime achievement awards from dental academies and institutions.

Throughout his career, Dr. Dorfman has been committed to educating the public about the world of dentistry and to giving back to the community. Dr. Dorfman and Discus Dental, Inc., together with the Crown Council of Dentists, an alliance of dentists throughout the United States and Canada, have raised and donated more than $20 million to more than 115 children's charities, including St. Jude's Children's Research Hospital, the Children's Dental Center, and Garth Brooks's Teammates for Kids Foundation.

Dr. Dorfman has been a repeat judge for the Miss South Carolina, Miss Oregon, and Miss Louisiana USA beauty pageants. He loves to water and snow ski, bike, climb, swim, and scuba dive, and maintains a vigorous workout schedule. Residing in Beverly Hills, California, he is an aspiring photographer and "wanna-be" musician and enjoys spending time with his three daughters, Anna, Charlotte, and Georgia, and his wife, Jennifer, Donald Trump's favorite "Apprentice."

Paul Lombardi

Paul Lombardi is an award-winning on-air television reporter and producer in New York City, with a master's degree in journalism from New York University. His work has appeared in the *New York Times* and the *Manhattan Spirit*. On television he has covered politics, health, and entertainment for New York 1 News, E! Entertainment, and Extra. He has also appeared on CNN's *American Morning* and ABC's *My Kind of Town*. Lombardi has been a Tony Awards voter and a judge for the Miss Louisiana USA beauty pageant. He also writes screenplays with his brother Tom, and is working on a children's book about smiles with Dr. Dorfman. He lives in New York and California.